P EOLOGY

"Dr. Ava Cadell's book NeuroLoveology blends certain aspects of neuroscience with the science of love, offering mindful techniques to help grow more brain cells while growing an intimate relationship.

One of the biggest problems facing people today is an overwhelming number of distractions, both internally and externally, that make life balance almost impossible. NeuroLoveolgy gives people the tools to replace these distractions with mindful intimacy and regain passionate living.

There are several brain chemicals that come in to play during a relationship. Knowing what triggers their release is an important part of romance. NeuroLoveology helps to identify activities that release pleasure hormones so that you can effortlessly get into the mood for love."

– Best selling author of Men Are From Mars, Women Are From Venus and over 20 other books on relationships, Dr. John Gray

"NeuroLoveology is jam packed with helpful, useful information. Dr. Ava Cadell has given us a gift that keeps on giving. Lot's of wisdom, good advice, and tips for immediate transformation and a better future."

– Actress and superstar of ABC's General Hospital, Jacklyn Zeman

"Dr. Ava knows sex like Tiger Woods knows golf."

– National radio sportscaster, Jim Lampley

"My wife and I rekindled the passion we once had by following Dr. Ava's principles."

– Star of Grizzly Adams, Dan Haggerty

"Dr. Ava can tell you how to, why to, when to and where to. All you need to know is who to."

– Emmy Award winning Actor and producer, Alan Thicke

NEUROLOVEOLOGY

Print ISBN: 978-1-62467-171-5
eISBN: 978-1-62467-170-8

P

PREMIER PUBLISHING

Published by Premier Publishing
www.premierdigitalpublishing.com
Follow us on Twitter @PDigitalPub
Follow us on Facebook: Premier Digital Publishing

The author and publisher specifically disclaim any responsibility for liability, loss, or risk, personal or otherwise, which is incurred as a consequence, directly or indirectly, of the use and application of any of the contents of this book.

Trademarks: All terms mentioned in this book that are known to be or are suspected of being trademarks or service marks have been appropriately capitalized. Premier Digital Publishing cannot attest to the accuracy of this information. Use of a term in this book should not be regarded as affecting the validity of any trademark or service mark.

TABLE OF CONTENTS

This book is dedicated to anyone brave enough to fall in love.

ACKNOWLEGEMENTS

Peter Knecht, my husband, you have my heartfelt gratitude for your support and encouragement. I am blessed to have been married for 21 years to you and it is my wish for everyone who reads this book to experience the same kind of everlasting love.

NeuroLoveology would never have been possible without my amazingly talented editors Paula Tiberius and Shadley Grei whose contributions to guiding, shaping and polishing this book made my writing journey such a pleasure. I am an ardent admirer of both of your creative works. I hope that this project helps pave the way toward your own successes in whatever you pursue.

I'm thankful to my stepson Chance for his endless assistance to my needs with Loveology University, my blog, and all my social networks. Without your technical expertise, I would be in the dark, so thank you for showing me the light.

Thank you to Marilyn Calabrese for your diligent proofreading and for all the positive feedback.

Special thanks to my dear friend Dr. Ronda Fenn for introducing me to Dr. Swartz, a New York scientist entrepreneur, electrical engineer and inventor of the handheld barcode laser scanner. I am beholden to you both for that magical experience at The Swartz Foundation for Computational Neuroscience at UC San Diego where I was first introduced to neuroscience and the incredible researchers exploring the great complexities of the human brain. It was this unforgettable experience that inspired and motivated me to write *NeuroLoveology*.

I am so grateful to my spiritual friend Gurutej Kaur for introducing me to my publisher Hutch Morton, and I extend many thanks to bestselling author Dr. John Gray for writing *Men Are From Mars, Women Are from Venus,* and for all the other books on relationships and personal growth. Your personal endorsement for NeuroLoveology is a dream come true for me.

Last but not least, thank you to my hardworking publicist Jim Strzalkowski and Premier Digital Publishing marketing maven Julie Morales for promoting *NeuroLoveology: The Power to Mindful Love and Sex,* so that I can share my insights, helping people give and receive love all over the world.

FOREWORD

Love is a mystery and something we can always have more of. Dr Ava Cadell offers insights, techniques, and tips on how to have more love in your life – and more fun in bed!

"Dr. Ava" combines years of expertise from her extraordinary career as a Sexologist who has counseled couples with every sex and relationship issue imaginable, with research into the science of the brain. She shares many "mindful" sex techniques she has used in her practice that singles and couples can try for a much more interesting sex life. She explains the findings of her research into the world of Neurology and brings it into the realm of Sexology.

Culling over 100 brain "neuro-cises" that help your brain as well as your lover's to change and actually grow, she proves that the biggest sex organ in the body is the brain. By learning what the brain is doing, she demonstrates that we can create more thrilling sex lives by being curious and excited, relaxed but never bored. (And she discovers we can have "BrainGasms!") With a focused mind and an open heart, being more "mindful" makes sex more fun, and love more possible.

Anka Radakovich
Sex Columnist and Author of THE WILD GIRLS CLUB, Part 2
Skytower Publishing, Feb 14, 2014
New York, New York, 2014
Twitter: @ankarad

INTRODUCTION

NeuroLoveology is the blending of brain science with the science of love. I created this term to encompass all the fascinating discoveries and connections I've made between these two worlds, and to map out precisely how our minds tick when it comes to attraction, romance, love and sex.

Perhaps you believe that love should remain a mystery and that understanding the how and why will only diminish the extraordinary feelings of romance. On the contrary, by learning exactly what the brain is doing, we arm ourselves with the tools to create exciting sex lives, rewarding intimacy, and much more fulfilling romantic relationships. Our stumbling blocks are transformed into building blocks.

Recent advances in neuroscience have yielded astonishing data about how the brain is able to change itself, and how we can utilize this "plasticity" to our advantage. For me, the most fascinating aspect of these studies is the careful unraveling of the magic behind love and attraction. As counter-intuitive as it may sound, demystifying the complicated network of neurotransmitters can actually help us to feel even sexier!

Perhaps you are a businessperson who complains about not having enough time or energy for romance, or you're a busy parent who would like to be more focused in the bedroom. Maybe you are confused about why you and your partner are drifting apart, or you're single and looking for an exciting new relationship. This book will open your mind to receive the kind of love you desire right now and experience the kind of sexual intimacy that you always dreamed of.

You'll discover new ways to make your environment more love-friendly, mindful exercises to overcome daily distractions that prevent you from connecting to your partner, and many more exciting psychology-based tools to enhance your relationship emotionally and sexually.

I have included over 100 solo or duo "neuro-cises" (brain exercises) for singles and couples that will help you reach your goal, whether it's meeting your next potential partner, improving intimate communication with your current partner, enriching your relationship or deepening intimacy. All the neuro-cises are intended to expand your horizons while growing your brain cells. I have listed all of the neuro-cises in the index at the back of book for convenient reference.

I have also gathered over 100 valuable insights to share with you from the world's top experts in their fields, including Dr. John Gray, Dr. Helen Fisher, Dr. Deepak Chopra, Dr. Mehmet Oz, Dr. Daniel Kahneman, Dr. Daniel Amen, Dr. Louann Brizendine, Dr. Dan Siegel and many more. For their fantastic and inspirational quotes, look for this Brainy-Yak icon:

The material in this book is not intended to replace professional therapy, mental or physical treatment, but to provide a beneficial groundwork for personal growth based on my years of research, life experiences and development of self-improvement techniques. As with any self-help book, results will vary from one individual to another.

If you invest the time to explore this experiential, playful, hands-on book, I guarantee you will take away a love-changing experience that will last you a lifetime.

CHAPTER ONE
The F.A.C.E.S. of Love

Of all the facets of our mental, physical and emotional lives, love is easily the most complicated. Love is exciting, overwhelming, terrifying, excruciating, exhausting, and exhilarating all at the same time. It is a constantly evolving concept that never stops changing, despite the 'happily ever after' narratives our popular culture suggests.

"Love brings up our unresolved feelings. One day we are feeling loved, and the next day we are suddenly afraid to trust love," writes Dr. John Gray, relationship guru, global speaker and author of over twenty books including the bestseller, *Men Are From Mars, Women Are From Venus.*

While romantic comedies would have us believe that love has a beginning, middle and end – you meet, you date, you fall in love - I believe that the real love story begins after the movie.

Biological anthropologist Dr. Helen Fisher writes about the evolution of human sexuality, monogamy, adultery and divorce, gender differences in the brain, the chemistry of romantic love, and most recently, human personality types and why we fall in love with one person rather than another. She has famously identified the stages of love as lust, romantic love, and attachment or "We're strangers", "We're partners", and "We're family," which is an essential foundation. But what I've discovered in my practice is that this is just the beginning of the conversation.

As a Loveologist® with doctorates in human behavior and human sexuality, most of my work revolves around helping people give and receive love within the context of an ever-evolving relationship. Regardless of whether my clients are straight, gay, bi, curious, monogamous, monogamish, married, polyamorous, swingers, single, young, old, disabled or enabled, they all want to be loved. It has been my mission to teach the skills needed to make fulfilling love a priority, and along the way I've discovered that the secret to successful relationships has a lot more to do with what's between our ears than what's between our legs.

"A loving heart is the beginning of all knowledge."

– *Thomas Carlyle*

To decipher the "brain code" that unlocks the mysteries of passion, romance and happiness is to discover precisely how to find love and maintain it until the end of time.

Defining the Tools at Play

The first step in cracking the code is to identify the players: Brain, Mind, and Emotion. The brain is the organ in our heads that controls every function we perform. The mind uses the messages from our brains to interpret, reason, think and feel. Emotions are the mental reactions experienced in response to the interplay between the brain and mind, manifesting in a variety of physiological and behavioral responses.

Wait, what?

In other words, the brain is tangible, the mind is not, and as Raphael Cushnir, author of *The One Thing Holding You Back: Unleashing the Power of Emotional Connection* defines it, "an emotion is a message from your mind delivered to your body as a physical sensation."

The brain, mind and emotion are all interconnected. The brain is the delivery system by which messages are sent to the body, the mind processes these messages and applies appropriate emotions, and then that coded message is sent to the physical body for expression. Basically, the brain is the match, the mind is the spark, and the emotion is the flame.

While some of this happens consciously, a majority of this process takes place below the surface with the help of some highly potent chemicals.

Chemical Cocktails of Romance

Attraction works very much like a powerful cocktail. The process of getting '"turned on" through the feelings of attraction and desire is powered by various chemicals and hormones that complete an intricate recipe within your body.

If your brain is the bartender and your body the glass, these various elements are the special ingredients in the cocktail of life. While vodka can be fine on its own, you need to bring in the added elements of peach schnapps, cranberry juice and orange juice in order to sip a little "Sex On The Beach." The brain works much the same way. You may have one basic thought ("that girl is pretty"), and then suddenly with a splash of this chemical and twist of that hormone, you're giddy with desire!

Oxytocin is like the strawberry in the strawberry daiquiri. It is released by the pituitary gland and has been linked to the formation of close social bonds because it decreases stress levels and increases trust.

Vasopressin is like the tonic in the gin. It is a calming chemical secreted by the hypothalamus that fuels long-term relationship bonding.

Androgens are the Tabasco in the Bloody Mary. Testosterone is the primary sex hormone from a group called "Androgens." Produced mostly by male testicles, it can also be created in smaller amounts by the female ovaries. While most men produce 6 to 8 mg of testosterone a day, most women produce only 0.5 mg. Low levels of testosterone have been linked to decreased sexual desire as well as causing some men to have difficulty maintaining an erection, while high levels may increase sexual lust in both sexes. In fact, women in their reproductive years have seen their testosterone levels spike in the middle of their menstrual cycle, which helps explain why many women have reported an increased sexual appetite when they are most fertile.

Estrogens are like the cranberry juice in a Cosmopolitan. These are the sex hormones produced primarily by a female's ovaries that play a large role in the female body by stimulating the growth of sex organs, breasts and pubic hair, while also regulating the menstrual cycle. The brain of both sexes also produces estrogen, though what part this plays in male sexuality hasn't yet been established. It is believed by many researchers that it plays an important role in sexual appetite.

Nitric Oxide is the olive juice in the dirty martini. This chemical is released by the genitals during arousal. It increases blood flood to the sex organs, especially the penis.

Pheromones are the lime juice on the glass rim of a margarita. These scented hormones are found primarily in the odor-producing apocrine glands of the armpits and other areas of the body that have hair follicles. Linked to sexual attraction, research has indicated that we may select our partners by using a set of subtle smell cues, since no two people have the same odor print, with the exception of identical twins. However there is much research in progress about the exact way these hormones work, so the jury is still out.

Neurotransmitters are like the various fruits in sangria. Epinephrine, norepinephrine, dopamine, serotonin, and phenylethylamine (PEA) are the 'BrainGasm' neurotransmitters that stimulate motivation and drive. After playing a minor role in the initial phase of love, it is really in the second stage ("Adventure") that they take the spotlight and work to help the brain feel balanced. Epinephrine and norepinephrine are responsible for the feelings of an "adrenaline rush", with high levels associated with anxiety and low levels with depression.

The Iceberg Mind

No, I am not suggesting that the mind is responsible for the demise of the Titanic. Instead, I am using an iceberg as a metaphor for the two basic elements of the mind, the conscious and the subconscious.

Picture a huge iceberg poking out of the water, the gleaming white peak glistening in the sun. That peak is our conscious mind. This is where we think about food and sex when we are hungry or horny. We are aware of the thoughts in the conscious mind as they are happening. Then picture the massive chunk of ice below the water's surface getting larger and wider as it extends all the way to the ocean floor. This is our subconscious mind, which lurks below our awareness level, and stores everything that has ever happened to us. It allows us to retrieve our memories and emotions when we need them.

"The mind is like an iceberg, it floats with one-seventh of its bulk above water."

– Dr. Sigmund Freud

Amazing as it may sound, the conscious mind controls our brain about 5% of the day (that's like eating only one shrimp from a magnificent seafood buffet), whereas the subconscious mind has a hold on our thoughts the rest of the time. Imagine if we could access the full all-you-can-eat buffet and choose exactly what sustains us with the best taste and nutrition imaginable?

Under the surface of your mind, there may be submerged volcanoes about to erupt at any moment, but there may also be beautiful coral reefs, sunken treasures, and extraordinary marine life to be explored. It's important to become aware of the way our conscious and unconscious minds work together, because the life choices we make will either feed the dangerous shark or the friendly dolphin in the ocean of our minds. Which do you want to grow stronger, Flipper or Jaws?

How the Mind is Fed

I'm going to assume that most people would rather feed the friendly dolphin than the dangerous shark, but what does this mean exactly? What I'm talking about is learning to see the way the mind processes information and understanding whether this focus benefits or hinders personal growth.

Energy Guru Gurutej Khalsa, author of *Slice of the Beloved* and *The 13th Month,* outlines an easy way to understand the various thought processes with The Three Minds:

1. The Positive Mind is hopeful and believes that anything is possible.

2. The Negative Mind is protective and motivated by fear.

3. The Neutral Mind is calm and allows you to see everything that has happened to you (good or bad) in terms of gifts.

The Three Minds battle to control your every thought, and the winner of that battle informs your course of action.

If you're a surfer out on your board waiting for the next magnificent wave and you suddenly hear a nearby splash, your Positive Mind might immediately think Flipper has come to visit. At the same time, your Negative Mind is convinced Jaws has come to eat you for lunch. Simultaneously, your Neutral Mind wonders what caused the splashing sound, and turns, with no assumptions, to see that a gull has landed nearby by for a quick bath.

The Neutral Mind weighs the information offered to the Positive and Negative Minds with a quick resolve, steering you toward your best path.

Do you know how you would respond if you were on that surfboard? Would your immediate thought be "Flipper! Cool!" or "Jaws! Aaaah!?" Would you get into a mental war with yourself and succumb to a roller coaster of emotions, or would you allow your Neutral Mind to calmly guide you to safety?

Indian Philosopher, author, speaker and humanitarian, RVM, refers to this interplay of the brain, mind and various conscious levels as "The Thought Factory", suggesting that this factory is responsible for our emotional response to every aspect of life, both positive and negative. Love, hope, and compassion, as well as fear, jealousy and grief, are all produced by the invisible workers of our interior workshop.

> *"The Achiever says his Thoughts led him to Success and the Criminal says his Thoughts led him to Crime. Everybody thinks, but what we Think determines our Destiny."*
>
> *– RVM*

NEURO-CISE: SUBCONSCIOUS, SOLO

To attract a new partner, revive sexual interest in a long-term relationship or become a better partner, you need to send messages to your subconscious mind that will begin to create the love you want. For example, imagine if you allowed negative self-talk to dominate your mind, constantly sending messages to your subconscious that you're overweight, or that you need bigger boobs, or that you need more money to impress women. Your body responds with the emotions that match these thoughts - feelings of unhappiness, melancholy, maybe even depression or despair. Are these the body messages of a person who attracts love?

Then imagine taking control of your subconscious mind by actively sending positive messages to it. You look in the mirror and say, "Those extra five pounds look good on me," or "My breasts are beautifully naturally shaped," or "I have creative date ideas that impress women without costing me a lot of money." Now your mind responds with positive emotions that in turn create positive body messages. You are in attraction mode.

RVM also writes about "The Thought Chain" in his book *Power Your Life with PEP, Discover the Secret of Thinking and Living Positively All the Time!* We can use it to break our negative relationship habits and create new, positive ones.

It's exciting to think that we can gain control of our romantic and sexual lives by utilizing the complex inner workings of our mind and body that are happening anyway whether we guide them or not. Why not find love? Why not improve your sex life? No matter what stage of a relationship you are in, there are ways to guide your inner messages to bring about a better result. I'm not saying it doesn't involve work, but what is your happiness worth?

NEURO-CISE: THOUGHT CHAIN, DUO

The Thought Chain begins with a thought that leads to a feeling. If the mind thinks of a happy thought, we feel happy. Thus, the electrical vibrations produced by our thoughts create all of our feelings. If thoughts produce feelings, what do feelings produce? Feelings produce actions. So a happy thought leads to a happy feeling which in turn leads to a happy action. The next link is habit. Repeated actions create habits and this forms the fourth link in the Thought Chain. Now let's use the Thought Chain to create deeper intimacy in our relationship.

Think about a quality that makes your partner lovable, which will lead to loving feelings towards that person in your brain. Be sure to follow up with the action of giving them a hug and a kiss in the morning before leaving for work. Then at the end of the day, repeat this action, and repeat it again before you go to sleep. Now it has become a habit, guaranteed to enrich your romantic relationship and heighten intimacy.

The Emotional Evolution of a Romantic Relationship

Have you ever heard the expression, "The only thing that remains constant is change?" In my extensive work with all kinds of people in all sorts of relationships, this basic rule has proven true time and time again. I have witnessed countless stages of intimacy, romance, love and friendship, and have at last been able to group my findings into five areas. Building on Helen Fisher's three stages of love, I propose "The Five F.A.C.E.S. of Love."

F - Fascination

A - Adventure

C - Comfort

E - Energy

S – Success

Let's take a closer look at each of these phases to see what we can learn from each one and how we can enhance and improve our overall experience.

Fascination

The first stage in a new relationship is based around fascination with each other, the time during which we give off chemical signals that result in that infamous 'spark' that lights up all of our senses.

Under the spell of fascination, we might be tempted to do things outside our normal behavior because the feelings inspired by a new possible romance are exciting and fun.

 "Love is the master key that opens the gates of happiness."

– *Dr. Oliver Wendell Holmes*

It's like putting on a new pair of designer shoes for the first time and you love the way you look. You can't wait to wear them again and again. Or it's like test-driving an exotic sports car. Turning on its engine turns you on. You drive around the block a few times and run through the gears to see if it's a keeper.

We are all familiar with the feelings this fascination can ignite, but what exactly is this spark and where does it come from?

One scientific explanation is pheromones, chemical signals released by humans that send subconscious messages regarding physical attraction. Dr. Ivanka Savic of the Karolinska Institute found that the hormone-like smells "turn on" the brain's hypothalamus, which is normally not activated by regular odors. This is a very important finding because it identifies the stimulation of a specific area of the brain that is known to modify emotions, hormones, reproduction and sexual behavior. This can trigger curiosity in the brain as it works to comprehend these changes, thereby generating fascination with the person responsible for the internal shift. When we fascinate someone, we attract him or her, and they want to meet us, date us, make love to us and cease to think of anything else. People want to connect with us and when they do, they're more likely to fall in love with us!

Did you know that 80% of a person's initial impression of a potential mate is non-verbal? Yes, we can be fascinating without saying a word! The messages sent to others are communicated by posture and facial expression, which are universal. A smile is an open door of approval in any language, whereas crossed arms are a signal of unapproachability.

We must identify our fascinating qualities and use them to our advantage in combination with the body language of attraction. In a relationship, it is important to sustain confidence because even if the love doesn't fade, the compliments might. We may find ourselves in the position of upholding our own self-worth in the face of withering support in this area (which is something that can be worked on too, as you will see in coming chapters). Focusing on your strengths builds confidence and positive body language, just as focusing on your weaknesses makes you shrink and wither. It's not rocket-science, but it is scientific.

NEURO-CISE: PERCEPTION, SOLO

Single people need to be aware of their fascinating qualities because it creates a starting point for finding a partner, if that's the goal. By projecting an attractive image we create options for meeting potential partners. Our unique qualities are our calling card for inviting fascination. So ask yourself, "How do I want to be perceived by my partner?" For instance, if being health conscious is a strong quality, then time spent at a gym, yoga class, health food restaurant or health expo can create more opportunities for romantic introductions. There's nothing more attractive than a confident person who owns their strengths, and you have the tools to project this image – they're all in your head right now! Sending out the signals of interest amplifies the fascination radar and invites conversation. You can impact others to perceive you through your body language, your facial expressions, the sound and projection of your voice and your actions.

♥ Facial expressions are universal as emotions for happiness, sadness, anger, surprise and fear are the same across all cultures. A genuine smile can be contagious in the most pleasant way.

♥ Body movements, hand gestures and various postures communicate your confidence, insecurity, sexiness, inhibitions, self-love or self-doubt.

♥ Eye contact can communicate curiosity, attraction, surprise, fear, desire and love. It takes three quick glances followed by one three-second gaze to send a signal of flirtation in a public place. MRI scans of the brain have shown that eye contact activates the reward center or ventral striatum, so we are wired to interpret someone gazing into our eyes as satisfying.

♥ When you speak, your voice reflects your psychological and emotional state of mind. Verbal sounds are not just about what you say. It's also how you speak that impacts people's perception of you. The tone of your voice can entice or repel someone you wish to attract. You want to produce warm, cheerful, and gracious tones that convey your true personality and sincerity. Be sure to give a compliment followed by an open-ended question like, "That's a great jacket, where did you get it?"

♥ You can connect subconsciously by subtly copying the actions of the person you are attracted to in order to get into sync with them. So, if they cross their legs, follow suit but don't be too obvious.

Dr. Antonio Damasio, professor and head of neurology at the University of Iowa has found that the moment of attraction, in fact, mimics a kind of brain damage, where he has found that people with damage to the connection between their limbic structures and the higher brain are smart and rational but unable to make decisions. "They bring commitment phobia to a whole new level. In attraction, we don't stop and think, we react, operating on a "gut" feeling, with butterflies, giddiness, sweaty palms and flushed faces brought on by the reactivity of the emotional brain. We suspend intellect at least long enough to propel us to the next step in the mating game-flirtation."

Amp Your Radar

Here's another tip for singles: Take along a "flirting prop" such as a book or magazine (something that reveals your unique style or interests) so that people will be motivated to approach you. Or wear a flattering hat, T-shirt with a logo or carry a bag that has an eye-catching slogan. Borrowing a dog or a baby for a walk around the park is an immediate attention grabber and makes it easy for people to engage in conversation. But remember that the props you choose will affect how others perceive you.

During this introductory fascination phase of a relationship, we play and carefully reveal various parts of our personality, testing the waters, looking for signs that it's okay to lower our guard enough to move into the next phase.

Adventure

When fascination evolves to the adventure stage, the relationship takes off and we continue to explore new passionate territory. This is the phase where we can't get enough of each other, and both men and women are releasing the hormones testosterone and estrogen, which play a major role in sex drive. There's also adrenaline pumping during this time, which results in a sensation most commonly described as "madly in love." This description is less euphemistic than you think!

Dr. Fisher's research shows that when we fall head over heels in love, the ventral tegmental area gets fired up. This is the region that creates the natural stimulant dopamine, producing feelings of energy, craving and obsession. Our heart races and we feel butterflies in our stomach, which ignites desire with a rush of pleasure. The brain's reaction to a dopamine spike is the same as taking cocaine!

> "Romantic love is not an emotion. ... It's a drive. It comes from the motor of the mind, the wanting part of the mind, the craving part of the mind."
>
> - Dr. Helen Fisher

The adventure stage is comparable to a rollercoaster ride. We're up and down depending on the attention of that other person, sometimes we want to scream, but we also laugh, and we hold on tight.

How To Become 10 Times Bolder

The adventure stage inspires creative thinking. Don't be afraid to fully explore this stage and push your boundaries. After all, when your relationship moves to the next level, you'll be glad that you've set the tone for a bit of naughtiness. I've had clients tell me that their sex lives have become boring, only to discover that, objectively speaking, their sex lives were always boring! It was just the chemicals making them feel excited during the adventure stage. Of course, exploration can happen at any stage, but why not go all out during this heady time?

One way to inspire creative thinking is to ask one question: What would we do if we were ten times bolder to be more adventurous in this relationship? Get a massage together? Read or watch erotica? Take up dancing? Make love in new places? Explore sexual limits with role-playing?

Ultimately, the best way to be more adventurous is to explore beyond comfort zones, push boundaries and embrace the unfamiliar by welcoming new uncharted territory. Not only will this add incredible new experiences to the adventure of your life but it will also help grow new brain cells and aid in the transition to the next romantic phase.

Comfort

As the relationship grows into the Comfort stage, many couples misread their feelings as "falling out of love" when, in reality, they are moving into a deeper, habit-forming love. While the stages of Fascination and Adventure are heavily based in lust, it is here in the Comfort stage that true love begins to take shape. According to Dr. Fisher, the Adventure phase ("Lust" in her definition) can last anywhere from six months to seven years. So the transition between the Adventure and Comfort phases helps to explain the seven-year itch!

Your partner has now become "family." As a couple, you have settled into the comfort zone, and the relationship feels like a favorite cozy chair or a pair of warm fuzzy slippers. During this phase, the brain releases oxytocin, also known as the 'cuddle hormone.' Oxytocin generates a feeling of satisfying relaxation, delivering a steady stream of calm that replaces that crazy, electric passion.

A Concordia University study revealed that the portion of the brain that responds to sexual desire (the striatum) also responds to pleasures of food, perhaps explaining that "hungry" feeling we get when

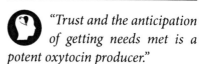

"Trust and the anticipation of getting needs met is a potent oxytocin producer."

– *Dr. John Gray*

we can't wait to touch our new partner. In contrast, the brain area triggered by feelings of love (the insula) is engaged in attaching value to the things that give us pleasure. This can explain why the sensation of love makes us feel rich.

As safety and relaxation replace spontaneity and lust, many couples feel that the relationship is coming to an end. Break-ups are common during this Comfort phase because often people are unable to redefine their connection to each other, or one partner has moved on to Comfort while the other remains in Adventure. I've often heard the phrase, "He loves me more than I love him," or vice versa, and sometimes upon further investigation, the truth is just that he's still soaring on hormones while his partner has moved on to fuzzy slippers. Difference of opinion over the current stage of a relationship causes strife, which can be smoothed considerably with awareness of the transition phases, and communication about creating passion.

NEURO-CISE: PASSION WHEEL, DUO

A fun and creative way to embrace the Comfort stage without giving up on Adventure is to create a Passion Wheel. On a large piece of paper, draw a circle (perhaps by tracing around the edge of a dinner plate) then use a ruler to divide the circle into 8, 10 or 12 pieces to create what looks like a pie chart.

Taking turns, each person writes one activity in a section of the pie chart that they believe will enhance the relationship. Continue to take turns until the pie chart is filled in. For example, you could write: talking, cuddling, kissing, caressing, bathing together, feeding each other, massaging, giving or receiving oral sex, making love in different positions and so on. Then each day, both partners take a turn choosing one activity to do together. This ensures that both partners get their needs met. You can also have fun pointing to an activity while blindfolded! Having your own custom Passion Wheel on display makes you both accountable for putting energy back into the relationship.

One couple I counseled was very surprised at the results from this exercise. The man didn't know his wife still wanted to make love once a week (they were only having sex once a month), and she had no idea he liked bubble baths. Creating a space and format for communication *about* passion is just as important as the passion itself! Of course there was further work to be done to figure out when this couple could actually find the time to make love and take baths, but once the motivation was there, scheduling was much easier.

It's amazing how often we leave our significant other in the dark about our intimate needs, and then blame them for not being able to read our minds. The security of the Comfort stage gives us a great opportunity to get closer to our mates and reignite the curiosity we're so busy assuming is gone!

Energy

Those lucky enough to reach the Energy stage are rewarded with a heightened union of intimacy that is known as Synchronized Energy eXchange (S.E.X.!) Having sex with someone that we're deeply in love with combines rewards from other stages, and also introduces a new hormone called vasopressin (the long-term commitment hormone) that is responsible for regulating territorial markings. Meanwhile oxytocin is still flowing, which increases empathy and communication, the key to sustaining a relationship long-term.

Experiencing true empathy with our partner means actually feeling the other person's sensations, movements and emotions inside us. This connection has also been identified scientifically as the articulation of mirror neurons.

Dr. Rizzolatti is an Italian Neurophysiologist and professor at the University of Parma in Italy who discovered special brain cells called mirror neurons in monkeys, hence the familiar phrase "Monkey see, monkey do." These mirror neurons work exactly the same way in human beings. They fire upon observation of an action or facial expression by another person, and 'mirror' the behavior in our own minds and bodies. For example, if you watch your partner licking an ice cream cone, you feel a 'virtual' version of the cool sensation on your tongue as well, or if you bump your head on the car door, your partner is likely to grimace and hold their head, too. Mirror neurons play a powerful role in understanding the depth of people's connection to each other whether it's through physical actions, speech, their minds or their intentions.

We can create mirror neurons to enhance intimacy in our relationship when we share emotions of love, happiness and even sadness. To create a deeper connection, share with your partner the things that are meaningful to you, and let them discover the meaning themselves. You can start with something as simple as a piece of chocolate! Let your partner watch as it melts in your mouth and create those mirror neurons that bring you closer. There are also many Tantric techniques that aid in deep intimate bonding, such as synchronized breathing and eye gazing. A deeper sense of commitment allows you to rediscover the sparks that first brought you together and it can feel like falling in love all over again.

Deep bonding energy is not only about reigniting physical urges. One of the most rewarding forms that relationship energy takes is the expression of gratitude. As the years go on, sometimes we forget those little 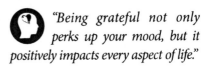 *"Being grateful not only perks up your mood, but it positively impacts every aspect of life."*

- Robert Emmons PhD.

"thank you"s that used to come so easily. We grow accustomed to our lives and fail to see the good in everyday occurrences, or worse, we fail to learn from things gone wrong.

Research on gratitude is piling up to show that gratefulness brings happiness. In his book, *Thanks! How the New Science of Gratitude Can Make You Happier*, Robert Emmons PhD points to studies that show practicing gratitude can increase happiness levels by about 25 percent. Not only that but it has several health benefits, including stress reduction, improved immune function, and lower blood pressure. Emotionally, gratitude fosters forgiveness, great self-esteem, generosity and cooperation.

NEURO-CISE: PERSPECTIVE, SOLO

Here is a great gratitude exercise by Marelisa Fabrega, author of *Daring to Live Fully* that can help put focus on all the positive things in life and make sure that the proverbial glass stays half full.

Obviously, things won't always go your way. However, gratitude isn't an emotion that is reserved for those moments when you get what you want. When things go wrong you can use the power of gratitude to release some of the negative emotions that you may be feeling due to the failure or setback that you just experienced.

After a negative event, put things in perspective by remembering that every difficulty carries within it the seeds of an equal or greater benefit. When faced with adversity, ask yourself the following questions:

- ♥ "What's good about this?"

- ♥ "What can I learn from this?"

- ♥ "How can I benefit from this?"

- ♥ "Is there something about this situation that I can be grateful for?"

Gratitude Journal

Starting a Gratitude Journal is a great way to acknowledge and appreciate all of the positive things in your life and to focus on what you have, as opposed to what you do not have. When you acknowledge gratitude, the law of attraction will bring you more of what you focus on. According to Dr. John Gottman, a leader on the subject of marriage, "Gratitude is the single biggest contributor to a flourishing marriage." It stands to reason that what works in the most complicated of human relationships works well in all relationships.

Buy a journal and take a moment each day to list at least five things for which you are grateful. For example: your health, the food on the table, the sun shining, your job, friends, family, pets and so on. Your daily gratitude will rub off on other people too, which will attract more potential partners, or take your relationship to the next level.

Gratitude Love Letter

Surprise your partner with a love letter. Put into writing how grateful you are for the gifts your partner has brought into your life. As more time goes into a relationship and the level of peace and comfort deepens, love can feel like second nature, so the magic of the connection can be taken for granted. By no fault of our own, we often most easily forget to acknowledge and compliment the person who has stood by us longer than any other.

Success

If love is the grand prize of life, then we can define Success by our level of satisfaction and happiness. Just the right levels of the mood enhancing chemical Serotonin (known as the feel-good neurotransmitter) are produced in the midbrain and brain stem, resulting in a profound sense of wellbeing, which is the goal of the Success stage.

When thinking about what it means to define a relationship as a success, I suddenly had this image of sitting by a campfire, making S'mores (for you readers who haven't been introduced to this delightful treat, a "S'more" is made of a marshmallow and a square of chocolate sandwiched between two graham crackers).

On our way to the campfire, our fancy shoes have been replaced by comfortable boots that were made to support a long hike. The sports car is now an SUV built to carry all the pieces of our life. The adventure has been the journey we have taken together to this campsite. The chocolate of addictive passion has become a comfort food. And we're wrapped up under the stars with the one that makes us feel safe and at home, no matter where we are.

It's important to note that you can have a successful relationship without realizing it. For instance, one of my clients came to see me because she was dealing with long-standing conflicts with her family. Her boyfriend, who was very supportive and loving towards her, would always accompany her and occasionally we would involve him in an exercise. One day while running through the list of things she would change about her family, I asked her what she would change about her romantic relationship and she realized that she wouldn't change a thing! She was putting so much attention on her family strife that she was completely oblivious to the fact that her romantic relationship was an incredible success, filled with love, friendship, trust, passion and respect. This revelation helped her put the focus on something positive which consequently gave her the ability to find closure with her family.

For a relationship to maintain its success, its partners have to grow together mentally, physically, emotionally and sexually. I think one of the key elements to accomplishing this is to continuously fall in love with our partner again, and one of the best ways to do this is to never give up the fun of flirting.

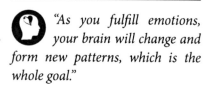 *"As you fulfill emotions, your brain will change and form new patterns, which is the whole goal."*

– Dr. Deepak Chopra

NEURO-CISE: FLIRTING, DUO

It may seem that flirtation ends once a relationship begins, but ideally it never ends. It is always important to remind your partner that they are attractive, smart, sexy and desired. Incorporating romantic reminders such as sweet notes, seductive poems, charming emails or thoughtful voice messages are great ways of flirting to keep a relationship new and exciting. There are many ways you can keep the flirtation alive:

- ♥ Leave love notes for your partner to find in his or her pocket, in their car, in the bathroom or imaginative place where they will least expect to find it.

♥ Record messages of love and appreciation in your most stimulating voice and put it in their car for them to discover on their way to work.

♥ Send compliments via texts to let your partner know that you are thinking of him or her.

♥ Plan a date night where you agree to meet in public as if you are strangers and flirt as if you're meeting for the first time.

♥ Make a flirty verbal request to meet at the foot of the bed and when you do, tell your partner what makes him or her most lovable to you.

Love is not a static emotion. It ebbs and flows, grows and changes as it evolves over time. There will be days when it feels like it is overflowing and there will be days when it will seem like it is dispersing. And as days become months and months become years, how the relationship defines love will change. The spark will become a flame. The flame will become a fire. The fire will warm the heart. And if both hearts are open, there's no end to the number of sparks it will find to keep the home warm.

NEURO-CISE: MISSION STATEMENT, DUO

As couples work through the various F.A.C.E.S. of Love, it can become challenging to remain focused on shared goals. Sometimes it can even be hard to remember what those goals are! One way to stay on track is to create a Couple's Mission Statement. Many successful businesses use a mission statement to keep the company focused on goals and ideals. It acts as a reminder of positive changes, growth, or advancements within the organization. If it works for big business, why shouldn't successful relationships be able to apply the same technique?

Collaborate to create a clear vision of shared principles and goals that can guide, encourage and strengthen the foundation of your union.

If you're married, use your vows as a starting point. Why did you choose to say those things and what do they say about your long-term goals as partners?

If you're not married but in a committed relationship, what key statements might be used to represent the shared goals for your commitment? If you're gay and in a state or country that doesn't yet legally recognize your relationship, this is also a great exercise for formalizing your commitment.

> "A great relationship doesn't happen because of the love you had in the beginning, but how well you continue building love until the end."
>
> - Unknown

And if you're single, what might such a mission statement say about the kind of partner you are looking for?

The Couple's Mission Statement might include:

♥ To love each other

♥ To help each other

♥ To believe in each other

♥ To wisely use our time together

♥ To be each other's best friend

♥ To respect each other

♥ To trust each other

♥ To support each other

♥ To be in love forever

♥ To be committed to understanding and forgiveness

♥ To remain loyal and encouraging without judgment

♥ To create a partnership that will grow mentally, physically, sexually and spiritually until the end of time

Building Together

Building a long-lasting and healthy relationship takes a lot of work, and one of the building blocks of this romantic partnership is mutual respect and understanding.

Part of this understanding comes from not only having a shared goal but also having a firm grasp on the way your partner thinks and processes information. Much discussion has been made of the different ways people approach life and nowhere is this discussion louder and more complicated than in the struggle to understand the basic differences between the male and female brains. At times it can feel like we are worlds apart while standing side by side. As it turns out, this is equal parts true and false. For some more insight, let's take a look at the next chapter on Why Male and Female Brains Clash.

CHAPTER TWO
Why the Male and Female Brains Clash

Much has been said and written about the fact that men and women think differently. They can see and experience the exact same thing and come away with completely different perceptions and feelings about a given situation. Many reality TV shows such as *Big Brother* and *Survivor* rely on this truth precisely because it creates so much conflict! But the conflict in your own relationship may not be so entertaining.

Even more fundamental than personality types, one fact is single-handedly responsible for this sometimes-painful conflict: women and men are literally wired differently.

He Thought, She Thought

Men chase. Women choose. That may sound stereotypical, but it's also true. The male brain is wired to dominate and to spread his seed, while the female brain is wired to nurture and select a mate that can give her the strongest offspring. We may be more intellectually advanced than our cave-dwelling ancestors, but, at our core, we remain the same.

In his best-selling book, *Mars & Venus Collide*, author and relationship specialist Dr. John Gray clearly outlines the evolutionary process that created the divide between male and female brains. While

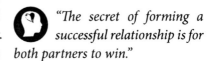

"The secret of forming a successful relationship is for both partners to win."

– Dr. John Gray

many jokes have been made about women's sense of direction (or lack thereof), the historical fact is that our male ancestors had to develop strong navigational skills in order to hunt and provide. Likewise, a man's inability to find something that is "right in front of him" can be traced back to the need for women to be hyper-aware of the details in their surroundings as they were left to care for the children while he hunted.

Dr. Gray further explains the physical differences in the male and female brain: "Men and women possess two different types of brains, designed equally for intelligent behavior. Men have approximately 6.5 times as much gray matter as women. Women have almost 10 times the white matter that men do. Information-processing centers are located in gray matter. The connections or networks among these processing centers are composed of white matter. These differences explain why men tend to excel in tasks involving gray matter local processing— like mathematics—while women excel at integrating and assimilating information from gray matter regions, required for language skills, because of their abundance of connecting white matter."

Additionally, research has indicated that women use twice as many words as men during the course of the day. Female social skills may have resulted from their smaller physical stature. While men could rely on physical strength during conflict, women learned to rely on their verbal skills. So the cliché of a talkative woman and a brutish man have less to do with stereotypes and more to do with the evolutionary skills developed in order for the human species to survive for thousands of years.

NEURO-CISE: WIN POINTS WITH HER, DUO

1. Make her coffee or tea in the morning, especially on a weekend.

2. Leave her a note saying you love her.

3. Plan a surprise picnic.

4. Give her a framed picture of both of you.

5. Hold her hand at the movies.

6. Be responsible for at least one dinner a week.

7. Tell her she looks beautiful when she gets out of the shower.

8. Do the dishes without being asked.

9. Massage her feet.

10. Thank her for loving you.

Portioned from Mars and Venus Collide, Dr. John Gray

NEURO-CISE: WIN POINTS WITH HIM, DUO

1. Allow him some alone time.

2. Learn something about his favorite sports team.

3. Compliment him to others so he can overhear you.

4. Be kind to his mother.

5. Tell him that he makes you feel safe.

6. Ask for his advice.

7. Surprise him with a sexy picture of yourself.

8. In public, flirt with him as if you're strangers.

9. Silently keep him company while he works on something important to him.

10. Initiate sex.

Portioned from Mars and Venus Collide, Dr. John Gray

Opposite Sides Of The Same Discussion

Have you ever noticed that when arguments arise, a man is more likely to take immediate action (leave the scene, stomp around) while a woman is often interested in sitting down and discussing it? This is because the male brain is linked more directly to the action centers, while the female focuses on feelings. By acknowledging this concrete physical evidence, our partner's reaction becomes less foreign, less inexplicable. We're more likely to give each other a break, knowing that corporeal factors are at play. If men and women want to have a consistently successful relationship and live together in harmony, then they must learn to acknowledge, understand and celebrate their differences, not try to convert their partner to their way of thinking.

Women sometimes complain that communicating with a man is like trying to talk to a tourist who doesn't know your language. Eventually, you resort to sign language. Men often complain that all women want to do is talk, talk, talk. It's

"During arguments, men need to ask more questions, and women need to talk less about their feelings."

– Dr. John Gray

important to understand that men generally use communication to share information while women use communication to build relationships. Most men are bottom-line oriented and will be better listeners if you get to the point quicker. They have a tendency to care more about WHAT is needed than WHY it is needed.

Also, as an action-focused provider, it is in the nature of men to offer suggestions to a partner's problem or situation. A man gets his dose of happiness from being a successful provider, so it can be easy for him to overlook the fact that just listening may be what his partner needs most. It's important to realize that a lack of emotional expression from a man does not indicate a lack of love.

While working to better understand the opposite sex, it's important to keep several key facts in mind:

♥ Men want to conquer while women want to nurture.

♥ Women want to be understood while men want to be admired.

♥ Men are more likely to focus on narrow issues while women see the "big-picture" from a wider vantage point.

♥ Women's brains are better equipped to divide their concentration on multiple tasks, while men can focus on specific tasks for long periods of time without distraction.

♥ Men can detach their emotions, relationships and information into separate compartments in their brains, while women are inclined to link them all together.

♥ Women are more in touch with the senses of smell, sound, touch and taste, while the primary sense of men is vision.

♥ Men are more likely to enjoy hearing graphic sexual words in bed while women are more aroused by romantic words.

♥ Female fantasies are usually tapped into something emotional and involve the whole person or couple engaged in kissing, foreplay and lovemaking. Male fantasies are usually more primal, include images of sexual body parts, and focus on orgasm.

♥ Modern man still has the innate programming from his caveman era to hunt and spread his seed while women are more monogamous. (Of course men have come a long way and we love them for that.)

Louann Brizendine, M.D. has written two extraordinary books on the battle to understand the sexes. *The Female Brain* and *The Male Brain* offer extensive insight into the different ways men and women are hardwired. Her studies show that when it comes to the brain, size really does matter. With larger brains, men literally think about sex more often than women. In fact, males have double the brain space devoted to sex as females.

In my practice, I'm often asked why men like to watch porn. As it turns out, there is at least one scientific reason.

There is a small almond-shaped segment of the brain known as the amygdala. Located toward the front on both sides of the brain, this area is at its most basic, the 'responder.' It operates differently in men and women, with the right side more active in men and the left side more active in women. Given the right side has more connections from the amygdala to the visual cortex, men are fundamentally more reactive to visual stimuli than women. Thus, the sight of a naked woman turns them on.

> *"Just as women have an eight-lane superhighway for processing emotion while men have a small country road, men have O'Hare Airport as a hub for processing thoughts about sex whereas women have the airfield nearby that lands small and private planes."*
>
> *– Louann Brizendine, M.D.*

On the flip side, a woman's amygdala is more directly linked to regions of the brain associated with internal awareness. Scientists believe this developed as a way to protect the body during pregnancy. This hyper-sensitivity to physical and emotional details creates a need to understand the "full story." Perhaps this is one reason why erotic literature is considered "female porn."

A Kiss Is More Than A Kiss

Studies have shown that the details of a first kiss are more memorable than the details of any other "first time" experience, including a first sexual experience. In her book *The Science of Kissing*, biologist Sheril Kirshenbaum explains the impact of kissing as being something we are wired to associate with positive emotions from birth: "When an infant is born, his or her first experiences of love and comfort and security usually involves some kind of kissing."

In adulthood, a passionate kiss causes our blood vessels to dilate and our brains receive an increase in oxygen. As our heart rate increases, our breathing becomes irregular, our cheeks flush and our pulse quickens. The pupils in the eye also dilate, which may be one reason why we close our eyes. The kiss also ignites a mix of positive neurotransmitters, including endorphins, dopamine, serotonin, adrenaline, and the "love hormone" oxytocin. These hormones are an important part of "keeping the love alive", which is why kissing more often is a surefire way to rediscover the spark in a relationship.

For a woman, a kiss helps determine the suitability of a partner via his hormonal markers. Women have a stronger sense of taste and smell, and kissing gives the best opportunity to get a sample. Kirshenbaum goes on to say, "It is nature's ultimate litmus test."

For men, open mouth kissing enhances testosterone through the exchange of saliva. Women receive a spike in testosterone as well, which increases libido. These findings are supported by a report led by Gordon Gallup at Albany University in New York that found, "the men surveyed overwhelmingly described kissing as a means to a sexual end whereas women reported that kissing allowed them to gauge how a prospective partner felt about them and whether the relationship was worth pursuing."

NEURO-CISE: KISSING, DUO

And where can you kiss your partner? The options are limitless. While the mouth is the most obvious, using your lips for a full body exploration of your partner is a tour worth taking:

- ♥ **Forehead:** Hold your partner's head with both hands and slowly kiss the spot right above the brow bone in the middle of the forehead with tender lips that form the letter O. This is a very intimate gesture and is also known as kissing the third eye, the gate that leads to higher consciousness in spirituality.

♥ **Nose:** One of the friendliest of all kisses is a gentle kiss on the tip of the nose. To make it more intimate, look your partner in the eyes at the same time.

♥ **Neck:** Tease your partner by moving your tongue and lips gently up and down, around the front and the back of the neck and end with gentle nibbling to give them shivers of pleasure.

♥ **Palm:** Kiss the palm with loose lips and slyly close their hand after, as if they are holding your kiss in their palm for safekeeping.

♥ **Navel:** Tickling the rim around the navel feels kinky and fun. Vary speeds and strokes to change sensation and top it off with a circle of smooches or a tongue that penetrates the navel.

♥ **Stomach:** Wet, open-mouthed kisses on the stomach can get a person's juices flowing. However, many people can be self-conscious of their stomach, so soft and sincere kisses all over can be just as good.

♥ **Spine:** You can kiss up or down the spine followed by soft licking and cool breaths to give your partner exciting spine tingling sensations.

♥ **Buttocks:** Kiss you partner from cheek to cheek varying the speed and the strokes as you explore their vulnerable and sensitive backside.

♥ **Feet:** French kisses on each toe and licking in between and along their arch will put them in a foot fetish frenzy. This is also known as "shrimping", the act of toe sucking or licking for sexual gratification of both partners.

Foreplay Isn't A Game

Foreplay is an integral part of a great sex life, as well as a healthy and long lasting relationship. A male client once complained to me, "Women consider foreplay everything that happens in the 24 hours prior to intercourse, whereas men only count the three minutes prior to penile insertion." While he was being funny, I had to admit that he was partially right! As we've discussed, psychological factors greatly influence a woman's desire, while a man is more concentrated on the physical aspects. Her surroundings, attitude, and mental state play a much larger part than his in sexual enjoyment.

Dr. Beverly Whipple, a certified sexuality counselor, sex researcher and coauthor of the international best seller *The G Spot and Other Discoveries About Human Sexuality*, states, "Female sexual response may be much more complex than anyone ever guessed. Men tend to view sex like they do many other things - in a linear way. To them, a sexual encounter is like descending a staircase that leads step by step to only one endpoint: ejaculation. Woman's sexuality is more holistic and encompasses a much broader scope."

In the word "foreplay", "fore" indicates that these activities are the predecessor to a more important main event, but this isn't necessarily true. Foreplay isn't just a prelude to sex, but a process that helps to warm up the mind and body for what is to come, which may or may not be intercourse. And the second half of the word, "play", should take away some pressure and put the focus on fun and exploration. We get to just be with one another in the sexual sandbox and build something together. The enjoyment and laughter is what's valuable, so we need to make that the priority over trying to build the perfect castle.

> *"For women, the process of making love - the holding and the hugging and the tenderness - can be as emotionally gratifying as orgasm itself, and sometimes even more so."*
>
> – Dr. Beverly Whipple

Simple actions can take on fantastic sexual overtones. For example, kissing the fingers can become a tease for oral sex. When kissing a woman's fingers, you might spread her fingers as if you were spreading her legs, then lick in between each finger like it were the creases of her vagina. And with a man, you could take his thumb in your mouth from tip to base in erotic ways just like it was his penis. That's sure to make your desires and indications clear!

NEURO-CISE: FOREPLAY, DUO

Stimulate your brain and get your body in the mood for love by making a list of ten sexual foreplay activities, and then prioritize them in order of your level of arousal. For example: kissing, cuddling, massaging, sharing a bubble bath, romantic dining, feeding each other, role-playing, erotic talk, oral sex, or mutual masturbation. If you don't already know what turns you on, you won't be able to communicate your needs, wants and desires to your partner. So, sharing your lists will lead to some cerebral communication and erotic experiences.

Here are some more ideas for turning a simple act into foreplay:

- ♥ Make out by a window to make the neighbors jealous.

- ♥ Play strip poker with your wildest cards.

- ♥ Distract your partner from working too hard by seducing them with a passionate kiss.

- ♥ Get comfortable on the floor with some cushions and read a romantic or erotic book together.

- ♥ Share long shaped food, such as an asparagus, spaghetti or breadstick by taking one end in your mouth and giving the other end to your partner, then nibble your way to the middle.

- ♥ Have a gentle playful wrestling match. The winner gets to be the receiver of pleasure first.

♥ Brush your partner's hair.

♥ Use a rolling pin to give your partner a massage, front and back.

♥ Have a naked pillow fight with your partner and kiss them once they've lost the battle.

♥ If you're lucky enough to have a fireplace, smooch or make love in front of the crackling flames.

According to psychiatrist and brain imaging specialist Dr. Daniel Amen, author of *Sex on the Brain: 12 Lessons to Enhance Your Love Life*, "Women need to ask for what they want sexually, and must teach their men through repetition, practice and good coaching."

Foreplay starts in the brain so take advantage of creative thinking and you'll have a romantic relationship that lasts.

Intimacy is Key

The thing about foreplay is that it can sometimes be more intimate than intercourse, which seems to focus on the end goal of orgasm rather than the immediate connection between partners. While foreplay can go on for hours, intercourse does not. Though it may not be a popular thing to say, I believe many people actually prefer foreplay to intercourse because it's much more relaxed and there is less pressure placed on performance. It's more about the other person than the orgasmic self.

There are four types of intimacy that should sound familiar to you, whether they're working successfully in your current relationship or not.

Cognitive intimacy is when a couple is able to communicate their basic wants, needs and doubts in an open, honest and comfortable way, without fear of judgment or rejection. This is a fundamental building block for relationships since couples who can't communicate their basic needs to each other usually don't end up getting what they want, which inevitably derails the love train.

Experiential intimacy occurs when a couple is actively involved in doing something they enjoy doing together, whether it's dancing, cooking, painting or gardening. They are literally interacting mentally, physically and emotionally.

Sexual intimacy can be a slow burning passion that includes a variety of activities such as caressing, kissing, erotic talk and oral pleasure that may or may not lead to sexual intercourse. Sexual intimacy can also include a broader range of sexual behavior such as anal play and role-playing. As long as both partners want to express their sexuality together, there is no right or wrong way to experience sexual intimacy.

Emotional intimacy is brought about through willingness, reciprocity, candor and experience, all of which are paramount for establishing trust necessary to bond with someone at such a deep level. To experience emotional intimacy you must first surrender to yourself so that you feel complete, then surrender to each other to complement each other's souls. Even if you struggle to express your feelings, you can work towards letting down your defenses and opening up your heart. Begin by listening with empathy and understanding, even when discussion turns to boundaries and relationship "deal breakers."

Intimacy can open up a Pandora's Box of feelings, so be prepared for uncomfortable feelings along with your feelings of pleasure when you release and surrender yourself completely to each other. It is often harder for a man to surrender than for a woman because some men are unable to distinguish the difference between weakness and emotional surrender, and they feel it's unmanly to be weak. It's worth learning the difference! That vulnerability you feel will enable you to merge into oneness with your partner. We all have fears based on past relationships, but without taking the risk of surrender, there can be no true love and intimacy.

Ultimately, we strive to open our emotional doorways to all of our senses, so that we can be present and emotionally available to one another. Intimacy is not just sex, but incorporates trust, comfort, safety, surrender, respect and open communication. Both partners must have a clear intention of fullness in the moment rather than being goal oriented. Think of intimacy like an artichoke. You have to peel off the layers and savor them before you can devour the succulent tender heart.

The key hormone in acts of intimacy is oxytocin because it is partially responsible for recognition, attachment, bonding and the building of trust. One of the neat things about oxytocin is that you can get your fix anywhere at any time. All you need to do is simply hug someone! The simple act of bodily contact will cause your brain to release low levels of oxytocin — both in yourself and in the person you're touching. There's even evidence that simply gazing at someone will do the trick — or even just thinking about them. Studies have shown that a rise in oxytocin levels can relieve pain — everything from headaches and cramps to overall body aches. Oxytocin has been observed to reduce the stress hormone cortisol in the body and lower blood pressure.

"Among men, sex sometimes results in intimacy; among women, intimacy sometimes results in sex."

- Dame Barbara Cartland

I've had many women tell me how annoyed they are that their male partner falls asleep after sex, but there's an excellent explanation. After an orgasm, men experience decreased activity in the prefrontal cortex, which is the region of the brain associated with processing and responding to information. Dr. Serge Stoleru published research entitled *Neuroscience & Biobehavioral Reviews,* where he reported that immediately following this reaction, two other brain areas (the cingulate cortex and amygdala) direct men to disengage from sexual thoughts. As if that weren't enough, men also receive a spike in serotonin, prolactin and oxytocin levels at this time, leaving them with a powerful sleep-inducing one-two punch.

Intimacy is a vital part of a relationship and it is intention that helps us to reach our goals. Without intention there is no focus or follow through. With shared intention comes a deeper heart connection and an even higher level of sexual satisfaction.

NEURO-CISE: INTIMACY, DUO

- ♥ Share all the qualities that you love about each other mentally, physically, emotionally and sexually.

- ♥ Share three strengths plus three things you would like to improve in the relationship.

- ♥ Share your physical, emotional and sexual boundaries without any judgment.

- ♥ Share three of your most romantic memories with each other and plan to reenact one that you both agree upon.

- ♥ Begin describing a romantic fantasy scenario and let your partner add to it. Then take turns creating additional scenes that get more and more erotic.

In some ways, intimacy works as a safety net in a relationship. At the core of intimacy is a genuine kindness felt toward a partner, which is of the utmost importance when challenges come up. What if, though, the challenge is, "it" won't come up at all?

His Challenge: Oh No, E.D.

Gentlemen, though it likely doesn't relieve the stress in the moment, you can take comfort in knowing that at least one report states that as many as 75% of men experience erectile dysfunction (ED) at some point in their lives. (Spark, 1991).

There are many reasons that ED affects a man's performance, including:

1. Vascular conditions

2. Alcohol

3. Medications

4. Diabetes

5. Abnormal nerve function

6. Hormone deficiency

7. Removal of the prostate gland for cancer

8. Other surgical procedures

9. Peyronie's disease

10. Illicit drugs

11. Smoking and diet, as contributing factors

The physical limitations of ED can create anxiety in men, causing a cyclical loop of physical and psychological symptoms. For example, if a man experiences a problem with an erection during one of his intercourse efforts, the next time he attempts intercourse the remembered failure manifests as a second episode of ED: a self-fulfilling prophecy.

There is an old school test to help indicate if the ED is a physical or psychological issue. Known as the "stamp test", perforated, non-adhesive stamps are wrapped around a man's penis before sleep to form a band. If the man is capable of having erections, the two or three that occur during REM sleep will tear the stamp band and suggest psychological cause.

There have been many advances in the treatment of ED, starting with the advent of the "little blue pill" (Viagra) and now expanding to several other brands including Cialis and Levitra. These drugs cause muscle relaxation, dilation of arteries, and blood inflow that brings about an erection upon arousal.

Given we live in a society where the expectation is for "real men" to be virile, confident and "alpha", it's often overlooked that they face many of the same insecurities and doubts as women. When performance troubles enter the bedroom, it can be a devastating blow to a secretly fragile ego, so partners should be cautious with any reaction, and take his lead.

Beyond erectile dysfunction, some men may feel a low sex drive. Almost as challenging as a lack of ability to perform, is a lack of interest in performing.

I had a client, James, who came to me concerned that his sex drive had diminished to a point that he wasn't even remotely interested in a sexual relationship with his wife. Married for six years, their relationship had started incredibly hot and heavy but over the course of the last year, he had lost almost all interest. Erections weren't the problem, but his desire to do anything with them was quickly becoming an issue in their marriage.

The first thing I had James do was see his doctor for a full checkup and have his testosterone levels checked. When that came back normal, we began investigating what was happening in his mind that may be influencing his lack of lust. At 36 years old, everything seemed to be going well. He enjoyed his job and maintained a comfortable level of success. He had a good circle of friends and hadn't experienced any serious life changes recently. His physical health was actually above average as he was training for his first triathlon! He talked lovingly about his wife and shared her desire to have children, though his lack of sexual appetite seemed to making that goal feel further and further away.

Honestly, the more we talked the less insight I had into what might be causing his troubles. That is until I invited his wife, Carol, in to discuss how his problems were challenging their relationship.

Though a lovely young woman, Carol spent nearly the first hour of our conversation listing everything wrong with their relationship and how James continued to let her down. As I listened to her unload her frustrations, I watched James respond to her. He nodded in agreement but also seemed to shrink next to her. The more she talked, the less he looked at me.

She wasn't being vicious, and held his hand as she spoke with tears in her eyes. It wasn't until she paused to wipe away her tears that I asked her if she still loved her husband.

She looked at me as if I were crazy and said, "Of course."

I then turned to James and asked him to tell me about the last time Carol had given him a compliment. He stared at me for a long time before he simply shrugged and said, "I'm not sure she likes me anymore."

Carol's response to this was to add it to the list of flaws she had spent an hour outlining. When I pointed out that I hadn't heard a single compliment toward her husband since she had arrived in my office, she replied that she thought she was here to discuss what was wrong, not what was right.

James actually cracked a small smile and said, "I know what's wrong. Everything."

What's interesting is that his half-joke inspired her to argue back with a list of things that were going right. Carol told him how amazing he was at his job, how dedicated he was about getting in shape for the triathlon and how her friends were constantly blown away by his kindness, generosity, and support of her own goals.

He listened to her rattle off all of his good qualities and then took her hand and said, "Thank you."

While there might be physical or psychological problems at the base of decreased sexual desire that can only be treated with medical attention, there are also many factors to examine in terms of everyday life and personal relationships that will give us clues as to how to reignite sexual interest. James simply needed validation, and he wasn't getting it.

Realizing this was a huge turning point for James and Carol. They left this breakthrough session looking like friends again. In their follow up session, when I asked if things had improved in the bedroom, they both giggled and blushed, nodding like a couple of kids who had been caught doing something naughty.

A feeling of success is important to a man's wellbeing. Having a partner that expresses trust, acceptance and appreciation helps men to maintain a healthy level of testosterone. Stress and depression deplete testosterone, so it's important to do an honest life evaluation of what's going on outside the bedroom.

NEURO-CISE: TESTOSTERONE, DUO

Here are some activities from my book, *The Sexy Little Book of Sex Games* that can stimulate testosterone:

- ♥ **Competition:** Your relationship is the ultimate in teamwork and a little friendly competition can be healthy especially when it leads to lovemaking. This game is called *Disrobing Desire.* See how long it takes each of you to slowly disrobe each other and appreciate every new area of skin that gets exposed, teasing as you go to create incredible sexual anticipation. Kiss, caress, and nibble sexual and nonsexual areas as you give compliments to each other. Whoever takes the longest to disrobe is the winner.

- ♥ **Setting deadlines:** Set your timer for two minutes and then have a *Tickle War* as you tickle each other's armpits, bare feet, ribs and tummy until the alarm goes off. You'll both be winners as laughter releases chemicals that trigger happiness and is infectious bonding couples together.

♥ **Planning an extravagant date:** Rent a limo for the night and bring along a bottle of a bubbly, fresh strawberries dipped in chocolate, and set the mood with sexy music. If you tell the limo driver that you're celebrating a special event, he or she will leave you two alone. Now that you've got your privacy you can truly enjoy the ride making out in that big, back seat like a couple of celebrities. But don't stop there, get your money's worth and go out for dinner followed by dancing while your *Love Limo* waits to take you back home.

♥ **Animal Magnetism:** Get into an animal posture and attitude by making the sounds and movements of your chosen animal. You can be a snake and slither all over your partner, a monkey playfully exploring him or her, a cat that snuggles, or any other animal you choose. If your partner guesses the animal you are, then he or she gets to choose what kind of animal he wants you to be in bed.

♥ **A Quickie:** For men quickies can be very exciting and satisfying and as long as the woman's mind is aroused, her body will follow. Having a quickie in a new place that is off limits can heighten the experience and raise the libido even more by releasing dopamine and testosterone.

If sex in a public place is your fantasy, here are some tips on how and where to make it a reality, though you may want to take along the number of a good criminal defense attorney, just in case you get caught and arrested for indecent exposure!

♥ **A shopping mall.** Try sneaking into the public restroom or a dressing room when the coast is clear, but look out for the public cameras.

♥ **On a train.** Take the train at night when it's on the last stop and find an empty train car, then snuggle up under a big blanket and have a quickie in spooning position.

♥ **Coat Check.** Whether it's at a formal wedding or fancy hotel, there's usually enough room and plenty of time to hide behind the coats for a quickie before people want to leave and ask for their coats back.

NEURO-CISE: TESTOSTERONE, SOLO

♥ Watch your favorite sports team. The good news is that your testosterone will spike if your team wins, but the bad news is that it will decline if they lose.

♥ Exercise increases your natural levels of testosterone so if your team loses, go to the gym and lift some weights. Testosterone levels are at their highest 48 hours after weight lifting.

♥ Sunlight exposure can increase your testosterone, but you only need about 20 minutes to raise levels, so don't bake your body, as sunburn is bad for you.

♥ Masturbation is good for your health and your testosterone levels, so be good to yourself.

Her Challenge: Coming Undone

Men aren't the only ones to face performance anxiety, though for many women the anxiety stems more from something mental than physical. Imagine if you will, having the tickle in your nose but never being able to sneeze.

Most sexual encounters involve a man's orgasm (if a man is involved), but many women find it challenging to reach orgasm. In fact, according to a study by Dr. Robert W. Birch as published in Pathways to Pleasure, 10 to 15 percent of American women have never experienced an orgasm.

> *"A woman's greatest challenge is to begin caring for herself as much as she is caring for others."*
>
> *– Dr. John Gray*

I know this to be true in my practice, where I've had many women come to me with this problem. It's sad to realize that the medical industry has treated a man's inability to get an erection as an emergency while no urgency has ever been placed on female sexual satisfaction.

With the advent of Viagra, there was briefly a surge of interest in finding something similar to increase female sexual desire. However, this search was a bust, mostly because it ignored the main issue. Viagra (and its ilk) don't increase sexual pleasure or sex drive, they simply drive blood to the penis.

Some of the many reasons that women are unable to reach orgasm are much more complicated than lack of blood flow to the clitoris.

Here are 15 orgasm barriers for women:

1. Traumatic past sexual experience
2. Feeling guilty about sex
3. Fear of pregnancy
4. Fear of failure
5. Fear of rejection
6. Lack of stimulation
7. Low self-esteem
8. Being too inhibited
9. Poor communication
10. Chronic tiredness
11. Resentment towards partner
12. Illness or Surgery
13. Medication or Alcohol
14. Pelvic Floor Prolapse
15. Stress

Getting to the bottom of any of the above issues will increase her desire, removing the psychological obstacles holding her back. Communication is key here. If you aren't willing to share your fears or inhibitions with your partner, you are limiting yourself to sexual frustration or "okay" sex at best.

Out of the women that do experience orgasm, only 17% report reaching a climax during intercourse. This is due in large part to the fact that sexual penetration does not usually stimulate the clitoris, which is a major component in female arousal. One way for a woman to increase the possibility of orgasm during intercourse is to simultaneously stimulate the clitoris through touch or toys. Keep in mind that the clitoris contains over 8,000 nerve endings — double the number in the head of the penis! So even an indirect touch with fingers or a vibrator can set "The Big O" in motion.

Many women assume a submissive or passive role during sex and find it uncomfortable to be too vocal with their own needs. It's important for both male and female partner's to keep this in mind and make a conscious effort to get her comfortable enough to express her own sexual needs. And, women, if you want to reach that orgasmic peak, don't be afraid to ask for whatever you need to get you there! Chances are he'll be relieved and excited to hear all about it! A good way to start is to assume a position with the woman on top. This allows her to control the movements and by leaning in various directions she can find the suitable clitoral stimulation.

One of my clients found an interesting way to rediscover her orgasm after having a baby. Janine was a 39-year-old mother of two who came to me with concerns that "her children stole her orgasm." Highly sexual and at times multi-orgasmic while in her 20's, Janine hadn't been able to achieve an orgasm in seven years, since the birth of her first child.

As we talked I learned that she had been a dancer for most of her life until she became a mom and her strength and flexibility had added much fun to her bedroom antics. What we discovered together was that she was self-conscious about the way her post-birth body looked, with stretch marks and added weight. Her husband said he found her more beautiful than ever, but the dancer in her mind didn't agree.

When I suggested that Janine blindfold her husband during sex, she laughed until she cried. They were not "those kind of people," but when I explained that part of her issue seemed to be with her body image, and that if she removed his ability to see her, she would be free to experiment and move around without fear that he was looking at the parts of her that she didn't like, she said she'd think about it. But she remained doubtful that she could find the nerve to bring it up with her sweet but reserved husband.

Well, she obviously brought it up because her husband insisted on coming to the next session where he greeted me with a huge hug and a bouquet of flowers!

Going back to what we learned about the plethora of white matter in the female brain making endless connections to information centers, we can extrapolate that women allow many other factors to seep into their sexual experience that may have nothing to do with sex at all. This is exactly what had happened with Janine. Her self-conscious body image about what childbirth had done to her dancer's body had interfered with her ability to orgasm!

NEURO-CISE, OXYTOCIN, DUO

Let's not forget about oxytocin, which is incredibly important to female pleasure! Some things that have been shown to stimulate oxytocin include:

- ♥ Collaboration: Holding hands, cuddling, eye gazing, synchronized breathing or listening to music together are all activities that build trust and release oxytocin for a woman.

- ♥ Shared responsibility: Parental bonds from breastfeeding a baby or nurturing an infant by holding singing or bathing him or her can release this love hormone.

- ♥ Being served a home-cooked meal: When a man can cook and serve a meal to his partner, even if it's just breakfast in bed, it makes her feel loved, valued and appreciated.

- ♥ Massage: Receiving a massage can be relaxing, healing or arousing depending upon the intention, but all of them naturally increase oxytocin levels.

♥ Breast massage: Gentle breast stimulation encourages blood circulation for a healthy lymphatic system and releases oxytocin. You can use massage oil or cream depending upon your partner's preferences. Begin by using light pressure in circular motions with your right hand on her left breast, then your left hand on her right breast. Follow by using both of your hands on each breast with gentle strokes that cover the entire breast area from the underarm, over the nipples down to the bottom of her rib cage.

Breastwork is part of the tradition within Ayurvedic massage that originated in India thousands of years ago. Some of the benefits of Ayurvedic massage include blood circulation, strengthening of brain function, and a calming and relaxing effect on body, mind and soul.

The higher the oxytocin level, the better you are able to deal with every day stressors. For men, increased oxytocin levels also lead to feelings of love.

NEURO-CISE: OXYTOCIN, SOLO

♥ You can engage in daily activities on your own to release oxytocin by thinking about someone you love and trust such as a family member or even a pet. Yes, research has shown that pet owners experience increased oxytocin from the love they give and get!

♥ Compassion is linked to higher levels of oxytocin, so volunteering for a charity or being generous to people less fortunate will make you feel good about yourself and reward you with the love hormone.

♥ Laughter is the best medicine for depression and releases bursts of oxytocin, so go to a comedy club or see a funny movie.

♥ Listening to soothing music releases oxytocin, so listen when you are in stressful situations such as driving in rush hour or cooking for company.

♥ Go to a spa and pamper yourself with a massage, facial manicure or pedicure to trigger some self-love and oxytocin.

The Baby Brain

Aside from maintaining a great sex life, many couples prioritize raising a family. Having a child is a life choice that initiates a whole new world of chemical cocktails, sexual challenges, and barriers to romance. While trying to get pregnant can interject a new dose of dopamine and adrenaline – you're doing something new together! you're bonding like crazy! – once the pregnancy begins, it's important to be aware not only of the physical and physiological changes, but also how each of your brains is processing the experience. Having a baby can certainly bring you closer together as long as you have empathy and understanding for what new feelings your partner may be experiencing, and how they may differ from your own.

Pregnancy Brain

The primary "pregnancy hormone", human chorionic gonadotropin (better known as HCG), helps to stimulate the production of progesterone in the ovaries during early pregnancy. The cells that make it go on to form the placenta and, once the placenta is developed, it takes over producing the progesterone, as well as estrogen. This added surge of progesterone and estrogen contribute to wild mood swings as their abundance results in blocking the mood-stabilizer serotonin. The stereotype of the hormonal pregnant woman crying one moment and laughing hysterically the next has substantial scientific basis.

Studies have linked HCG to morning sickness, which is one of the physical hurdles to watch out for during pregnancy. Also watch out for migraines, which could crop up as a result of increased estrogen. Other side effects of carrying a child may include heartburn, fatigue, frequent urination and hemorrhoids – oh the joy of it all!

Mommy Brain

Once the baby is born, the breastfeeding stage releases huge amounts of oxytocin in the female brain, causing extraordinary bonding between mother and child. Any partner, on the other hand, may feel left out in the cold, as the new mother's breasts have suddenly turned into faucets, not the playthings they once were. Many women report not missing sex at all as their lives have become consumed with the endless diapers and feedings, and their "intimate needs" are being met by that new little person who only wants to gaze into her eyes for hours at a time! Even a partner who is extremely hands-on cannot physically understand the transformation that the baby-mama has undergone. But they can certainly be empathetic and create a supportive environment for increased communication, which isn't always the first instinct of new parents.

Katherine Ellison, author of *The Mommy Brain: How Motherhood Makes Us Smarter*, draws on cutting-edge neuroscience research to demonstrate that, contrary to long-established wisdom that having children dumbs you down; raising children may

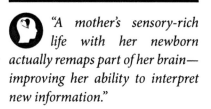

"A mother's sensory-rich life with her newborn actually remaps part of her brain— improving her ability to interpret new information."

– *Katherine Ellison*

make moms smarter. She benefits from enhanced senses during pregnancy and early motherhood, the alertness and memory skills necessary to manage like a pro, a greater aptitude for risk-taking, and a talent for empathy and negotiation. These advantages not only help mothers in raising their children, but in their work and social lives as well.

Daddy Brain

New dads are just as excited about the arrival of their child as new moms are, but they don't have the battle scars or the chemical cocktails to prove it. Or do they? Louann Brizendine MD, author of *The Male Brain*, has discovered that men do undergo hormonal changes during the baby's imminent arrival, and afterward.

The stress hormone cortisol rises considerably about four to six weeks after a man learns he's going to become a father, and begins to fall again as the pregnancy progresses. Brizendine posits that this surge of cortisol puts men into "alert mode", waking him up to the reality of the new life coming. "Get prepared!" his brain is screaming at first, and then as he creates and executes a solid plan, his brain chemicals calm down.

Dr. Mehmet Oz, TV Show Host and Cardiothoracic surgeon who has six *New York Times* best sellers including *You: The Owner's Manual,* and *You: Having a Baby* that he co-wrote with Dr. Michael F. Rozen, says, "Believe it or not, there is a very real thing called "daddy brain": Expectant dads go through hormonal and brain changes that roughly parallel those of their pregnant mates; it's why there are such phenomena as sympathy weight gain and sympathy pregnancy. Prolactin increases 20 percent in dads in the weeks before birth, and the stress hormone cortisol doubles in dads during pregnancy. Even testosterone dips after birth, allowing the male brain to let down its ultra-male guard and be receptive to bonding."

In It Together

As different as men and women can be, we all strive for the same things: love, respect, kindness, and personal growth. By understanding our differences, we are more easily able to focus on our similarities and the shared goals we are trying to build in our romantic relationships. And by focusing on the

"While men have little control over the physical course of their partners' pregnancies, they do harbor a lot of emotions about pregnancy and fatherhood, and thus need to be involved and invested."

- Dr. Mehmet Oz

desires we share, we will increase our levels of romantic and sexual satisfaction.

Let's take a closer look at some of these similarities by examining how the brain reacts to the explosive power of sex and creates a BrainGasm.

CHAPTER THREE
BrainGasm: Understanding the Elements of Love & Sex

In the 1980's, there was a commercial that used an egg in a frying pan as a metaphor for the dangers of drug use. "This is your brain on drugs," we were told, as the egg sizzled away in a menacing fashion. I've always thought you could describe the heart in the same way, getting grilled as we try to maneuver the frying pans of romance.

Though artists may argue otherwise, we don't actually fall in love with our hearts, or with our loins. It's our brain that does all the work. However, how the brain processes these feelings of love can manifest in physical ways that cause damage to the heart, or in emotional and sexual ways that affect other aspects of life.

Attraction causes many little explosions in the brain as lust and desire grows between two people. There are some basic things to keep in mind as you watch your relationship blossom and change in order to maintain the excitement that first inspired you to come together.

The Ingredients of Love

In our quest for everlasting love, we seek to express more of ourselves and experience more of life in tandem with the right partner. Expanding our experience to include another individual allows us to enjoy life to its fullest, which is the ultimate gift of our existence.

Love has a high value in our culture because it is an investment that endures, and has the ability to grow if nourished. Love is a precious gift that we earn and, as such, is all the more dear to us. If an individual can achieve a wholesome self-love, then two people uniting in love can become a powerhouse. Every trial and tribulation they go through together is an opportunity to know, feel and express more love.

Love is not about making someone feel guilty. I am convinced there would be more love and less guilt if couples would communicate their needs and expectations more freely and openly. Knowing and accepting each other's capabilities and limitations gets you off the "blame-game treadmill." You can then negotiate healthy compromises, or at least a frisky give-and-take.

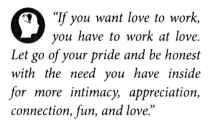

"If you want love to work, you have to work at love. Let go of your pride and be honest with the need you have inside for more intimacy, appreciation, connection, fun, and love."

– Dr. John Gray.

Love is not about manipulation and control. I can't think of a better line to express this than one spoken in the classic 1946 film *Claudia and David*, a tender yet honest look at a newly married couple. "Hold tight by letting go" becomes Claudia's credo when she realizes that marriage is more binding when neither partner feels smothered. Putting ironclad controls on your partner will only serve to alienate him or her, and your everlasting love will be in everlasting jeopardy.

Most of all, love is not a business arrangement; it cannot be bought. Let's be honest about the difference here. If two people enter a union out of convenience, or for financial or political reasons, that is an arrangement only. The situation does not carry the weight of everlasting love. And it cannot be expected to last or to become completely fulfilling. Everlasting love has no such price tag.

Love is not something you have one day and lose the next.

True Love Takes The Cake

If your relationship is going to evolve into something everlasting and true, you must be mindful of these necessary ingredients. While lust may be a cocktail (complete with loose inhibitions and a few headaches) love is like a chocolate cake. At its most basic, you can make a really rich, perfectly luscious chocolate cake with only five ingredients: chocolate, sugar, flour, eggs, and butter. Similarly, there are five elements necessary to make a really rich, perfectly luscious relationship.

Let's get out the mixing bowl and whip up some romantic love!

Respect

It is absolutely impossible to make a chocolate cake without chocolate. Without it, you would have to call the cake something else. I think of respect as the chocolate of a healthy relationship. Without respect, you can't have true love.

First and foremost, you must respect yourself before someone else will respect you. Just the way chocolate melts in the hot sun or becomes brittle in the freezer, your self-esteem and healthy ego undergo many challenges in life. Keeping your integrity and wellbeing intact will help you attract a well-adjusted partner who shows you the same respect you've come to enjoy from yourself. When it comes to love, your "measuring cup" of respect should remain as full as it was when you first met your partner, without wanting them to change. That's a good indication that love will prevail.

Respect can diminish over time, especially when you or your partner say or do hurtful things to each other. Whether it is verbal, emotional, or physical, abuse will kill respect. As I've witnessed in my practice, lack of respect is one of the most common reasons for the end of a relationship.

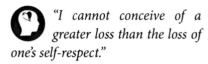

"I cannot conceive of a greater loss than the loss of one's self-respect."

– *Mahatma Gandhi*

Communication

Eggs work like the glue in a recipe, holding all of the other ingredients together. And the reason that the eggs are whipped with a mixer is that it gives the cake its light, airy texture. When the eggs are forgotten, the cake is left flat and crumbling. Likewise, if communication is left out of a relationship, there is little to hold it together, and joy is severely depleted.

Communication is like that secret ingredient that brings out the flavor of all the other ingredients. It creates a daily bond with your partner, whereby you can share your feelings, worries and happiness. Good communication can unleash strong creative energy between you and your partner, and with good communication, you can let your hair down and talk about anything.

Using powerful positive words like "love", "yes", "thank you" and "I'm sorry" can enhance your partnership and reduce physical and emotional stress.

Passion

Flour gives a cake its structure. It's the foundational ingredient on which everything else is built. Passion in a relationship works the same way. That all-consuming, euphoric, overwhelming, distracting, beautiful thing we call passion is likely what got you into your relationship in the first place, and it needs to remain present to keep things vital as the years continue.

Passion grows when you can be comfortable and uninhibited with each other, breaking down barriers with good communication. Passion fades when you have resentment, anger, or contempt for your partner. This is an area that cannot be neglected or taken for granted in a relationship.

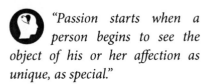

"Passion starts when a person begins to see the object of his or her affection as unique, as special."

- Dr. Helen Fisher

Keep passion alive by kissing every day to keep the juices flowing, recreating passionate memories and trying new and exciting activities together.

Trust

Butter gives cake batter its smooth texture and helps extend the life of a cake by keeping it moist. A smooth relationship with a long life is dependent on blending in trust.

I believe that people who cannot trust should not be trusted. Distrusting people are often deceitful because they imagine others to have their same fears and anxieties. One exercise I give my jealous or untrusting clients is to practice giving people the benefit of the doubt unless they prove otherwise. You cannot truly be connected to someone you cannot trust.

That warm, mellow feeling we experience when we trust each other is a large part of true love. Peace-of-mind in a relationship is vital to its stamina. And trust, like anything worthwhile, is something we earn over time, gradually, like the slow churning of creamy butter. Neurobiology research shows that when someone observes that another person trusts him or her, oxytocin circulates in the brain. The stronger the signal of trust, the more oxytocin increases.

Friendship

When making a cake, regardless of the flavor, one of the key ingredients is sugar. Without the presence of sweetness, it's not really dessert. Similarly, without the presence of friendship, it's not much of a relationship.

Friendship means being able to say anything to your partner because you have that ease of "best buddies." Best friends never take advantage of each other; they are there to help one another. Any good partnership includes the same love you have for a best friend.

Humans are hardwired to empathize because they closely associate people who are dear to them - friends, spouses, partners - with themselves, a new study suggests. "With familiarity, other people become part of ourselves," said James Coan, a psychology professor in University of Virginia. Protecting and helping others ensures our own protection and assistance. In serving others, we ultimately serve ourselves, creating a reciprocal loop of love.

NEURO-CISE: LOVE INGREDIENTS, SOLO

Think about the recipe of your relationship as I ask you these questions:

- ♥ Do you have all the proper ingredients? If not, come up with affirmations for each one that is missing in your life.

- ♥ Is the batter sweet enough or could you use some more sugar (friendship)? If not, create a weekly friendship ritual by spending quality time to empower and strengthen your friendship.

- ♥ Given the amount of butter (trust) you have incorporated, are things smooth, with a long shelf life? If not, work on building trust by being empathetic. This means doing your best to understand the world through someone else's point of view. Listen to them and practice random acts of kindness.

- ♥ How much more chocolate (respect) can be added? Let's be honest, you can never have too much chocolate! You have to earn respect and give it to receive it. So begin with unconditional respect for yourself by feeling it on a daily basis so that it becomes an automatic memory. Then accept others without trying to change them and they will respect you back.

♥ How much flour (passion) is required to give you the structure on which to build your ideal life? Find the passion in your life by doing what you love in and out of the bedroom.

♥ Did you remember the eggs (communication)? We can all improve our communication skills by thinking before we speak and listening to others without interrupting them. A powerful form of communication is called "Mirroring", which is repeating back what the other person said to you in your own words. Then, by asking if you heard them correctly, you will prevent any miscommunication or misunderstandings.

Once the cake is made, how does it taste? Start with the ingredient that is most prominent, the sugary sweetness of friendship perhaps, and add more of the other ingredients until you find the right recipe for you. Don't subtract some of the good things in order to counterbalance something that feels off. Why live with less chocolate when all you really need to do is add one more egg?

Don't forget to let your partner lick off your spoon. Remember, you're trying to make the perfect cake for two. Even if you're single, it's good preparation to have a good recipe ready to go for when you need it.

Building an intimate relationship can be a lot of fun. Like a dream job, the work doesn't feel like work when you love what you're doing and with whom you're doing it.

NEURO-CISE: PLAYFUL, DUO

Make time for adult play and jump-start your own sensual brainstorming sessions. It's good for the body AND the brain! "Scientific studies of longevity, medical and mental health, happiness and even wisdom," Dr. Siegel says, "point to supportive relationships as the most robust predictor of these positive attributes in our lives across the life span."

The supportive part is crucial. Loving relationships alter the brain the most significantly. Consider these fun activities:

1. Sizzle in the Kitchen

Most couples spend countless hours together eating meals over the course of their relationship. This is an area full of delicious opportunity! Take a moment alone or with your partner to evaluate how this time is spent in your current relationship. Do you grab sandwiches on the go and disappear into your respective home offices? Do you plan a thoughtful meal together at least once a week? Consider the fact that each shared meal is a chance to bond. How would you re-design your life to make the most of these occasions? While you're mulling that over, think about incorporating some brain-boosting foods to keep your grey matter happy and put you both in a good mood:

- ♥ Seafood (oysters, clams, sardines, crab, saltwater fish and freshwater fish)

- ♥ Nuts and seeds (particularly Brazil nuts)

- ♥ Lean meat (lean pork and beef, skinless chicken and turkey)

- ♥ Whole grains (whole-grain pasta or brown rice)

- ♥ Beans, broccoli and other fresh vegetables

- ♥ Blueberries

- ♥ Tomatoes

2. Shower Power

Take a hot, steamy shower with your partner first thing in the morning. The added company might be just the thing to get you going, especially for men who have the highest level of testosterone in the morning. So he may be eager to have sex in the shower. Don't worry ladies, research shows that showering will also give you an increased shot of dopamine that can trigger more creativity whether you have sex or not.

3. Spend the Weekend in Bed

Start by clearing your schedule. The only work you're going to be doing over the weekend is pleasing your partner between the sheets! Cook breakfast or brunch and then eat it together in bed. Order take-out food for dinner. Spending the weekend in bed should be both fun and intimate. If you have kids, hire a sitter to take them out and treat yourselves to at least a leisurely morning alone together.

4. Bathroom Bliss

Turn your bathroom into a pleasure palace. Turn down the lights and burn a couple of candles. A bathtub filled with hot water after a long, hard day may be just what you both need to unwind. Invite your partner into the tub with you. Enjoy the evening together and let the heat of the water and the intensity of the moment work its magic by removing all stress, replacing it with relaxation and sexual desire. Be sure to get out before the water gets too cold and before you get too sleepy as the decrease in temperature signals the brain to release melatonin (a hormone that is part of the human sleep cycle).

5. Unpredictable Quickies

Surprising your partner with sex in the middle of the day or night is a novelty that gets you both out of your routine. It stimulates the reward center of the brain, which releases dopamine and norepinephrine, leaving you both feeling satisfied. It also gives you a bonding *"Novelty is one of the key factors in driving brain plasticity."*

- Dr. Michael Merzenich

"conspiratorial" feeling that you're getting away with something, which creates anticipation for the next moment of spontaneity.

6. Passion Picnic

Create an outdoor feast! Take out a tablecloth, glasses, cloth napkins and a couple of candles. Include some aphrodisiac foods to increase romance, such as shrimp, asparagus, avocado, arugula, carrots, hot peppers, pumpkin pie and chocolate. Throw lots of pillows and a blanket on the ground and feed each other passionately. This is a perfect date idea for new partners, as the excitement will release adrenaline, the hormone that makes the heart race, mouth dry and hands sweat - so don't forget to take drinks and towels!

High Peaks and Happy Endings

The journey of taking a relationship from casual to friendly and all the way to intimate is to discover the best version of ourselves while building great memories together. As we work to build our history as a couple, it's interesting to consider exactly what the brain remembers.

In his book, *Thinking, Fast and Slow*, Nobel Prize Winner Daniel Kahneman shows us that the brain ultimately remembers only two aspects of an event: the emotional peak and the end. Consider that for a moment. While the minute details may be remembered with some effort, if you quickly recall the happiest moments of your life, don't you first zoom in on the highest peak of an experience? And isn't that memory balanced with the way that it ended?

Dr. Kahneman calls this "the peak-end rule" which essentially means that the lasting impression of an experience is most strongly associated with the peak emotional feeling and the final level of emotion at the end of the experience.

For example, perhaps you and your partner made love on the beach during your honeymoon and then picked up a shell to keep as a souvenir. You remember the high peak of making love, and the end gesture of picking up the shell.

Another high peak example might be surprising your partner with their favorite home cooked meal and the positive ending might be when doing the dishes together turns into a make-out session in the kitchen.

We often remember our sexual experiences in terms of high peaks and endings, too. Think back to the last time you and your partner had sex. What do you remember? The way your partner brought you a glass of water after your orgasm and cuddled up tight? Sometimes we let our sex lives drive on auto-pilot, not being mindful of our responses, our desires, or what really moves us. Examining what the brain is up to before, during and after lovemaking gives us some language with which to start the conversation.

Unmasking Sexual Response

We all know the logistics of how babies are made but how well do you understand what is happening between the first hint of foreplay and the last breath of post-coital relaxation? Dr. William Masters and Virginia Johnson originally postulated a four-stage model for sexual response, but I've created a model with five stages based on the knowledge and experience I've gained personally and from my private practice.

> *"Sex is an affirmation of life. By making sex a prominent part of it—placing it on the top of our list of priorities—it helps us face daily challenges in other parts of our lives."*
>
> – Dr. Stanley Siegel

NEURO-CISE: SEXUAL RESPONSE, DUO

The next time you have sex, pay attention to changes that take place and see if you can recognize these five distinct phases.

Phase 1 - Foreplay
The minute a man sees a sexy image or feels an intimate touch, his amygdala, which regulates his emotions, releases feel-good pleasure endorphins in his brain and triggers testosterone. These send messages to his body that he is getting turned on and make him feel sexually virile. His heart rate quickens and blood begins to move to the genitals.

Most women need to be prepared for sex with some foreplay ranging between ten and forty-five minutes. Whispering her name in her ear and then kissing her triggers the release of dopamine from the nucleus accumbens that will flood her brain with feel-good chemicals. Caressing her face, neck, shoulders, arms and other areas will increase her blood flow to her genitals and her entire body will become more sensitive. Her estrogen mixed with his testosterone increases their sexual desire.

Phase 2 - Excitement

Heavy-duty petting can take foreplay to a whole new level, especially when you know how it affects your mind and body. I like to call it "Love Play" as it is playful and can be a prelude to making love. It can consist of kissing, caressing, hugging and humping or stroking, all physical and psychological acts that lead to more sexual excitement.

Whether male sexual excitement is created by physical or mental stimulation, the result is the same. His blood flow is increased to his genitals and the penis begins to harden. Adrenaline actives the sympathetic nervous system, which increases his heart, pulse and respiration rate too. The ventral tegmental area (VTA) actually releases the dopamine, making him feel like a king.

Female sexual excitement affects the entire body with the increase of her heart, pulse and respiration rate. During this cycle, her breasts swell and her nipples become erect. Also, her vagina becomes wet. Like a man's penis, a woman's clitoris also becomes erect, up to three times its normal size. Her brain areas associated with the chemicals dopamine and norepinephrine production light up as they make her feel intense pleasure and excitement.

Phase 3 – Plateau

Oral sex is one of the most highly erotic, loving, and satisfying sexual activities you can indulge in that can lead to the Plateau phase, if you are not yet ready for sexual intercourse. Like any other sexual act, it all starts between the ears, so if oral pleasure is what you want be sure to communicate that to your partner because they cannot read your mind.

The head of his penis becomes engorged with blood and swells. For the uncircumcised man, the penis head pushes out of the hole in the foreskin. At the urethral opening, some men will secrete pre-ejaculatory fluid, more commonly known as "pre-come." This fluid contains semen, so wear a condom to practice all the necessary safer-sex precautions to protect yourself and your partner from STDs and pregnancy. The chemical vasopressin, a male counterpart to oxytocin is released to increase bonding with his partner.

Her body temperature rises and changes, which may explain why the face and chest get red when having sex. This is often referred to as a "sex flush" and with the increased blood flow to the genitals the color of her inner vaginal lips become a deep red. Her clitoris retracts under the clitoral hood. Her uterus is pulling upward into the abdomen widening the vaginal space allowing the penis to fit comfortably. The pituitary gland releases beta-endorphins, which studies show can decrease physical pain, including headaches.

Phase 4 – Orgasm
Many women say their best orgasms happen while receiving oral sex or when they use their fingers or a vibrator on the clitoris during penetration. The secret to simultaneous orgasms is to sync up your mind and body with your partner before having intercourse. Remember that an orgasm starts in the brain, so paying close attention to your partner's erotic cues will help you both reach a highly aroused state at the same time and maybe even have simultaneous orgasms.

At the orgasmic point, male blood pressure is rising and muscle tension is building to a peak as he's about to reach his orgasm. The testicles rise up close to his penis while his prostate gland is filled with fluid. The cerebellum controls muscle function as they contract involuntarily. When his pelvic muscular contractions begin, there's no going back, and the sperm shoots out of the urethral opening of his penis. His body movements during orgasm are totally unconscious according to brain scans.

In the female orgasm cycle, the uterus, anus, leg muscles, face and hands begin to involuntarily contract. Dr. Masters and Virginia Johnson referred to these muscle spasms as "myotonia" activated by the vaginal muscles. There are strong contractions in the vagina at 0.8 second intervals, the lungs are working at forty breaths per minute and heart beat can go as high as 180 beats per minute. While in the brain, a releasing agent called phenylethylamine (PEA), which is famous for being found in chocolate, makes her feel both physically and emotionally satisfied. A woman's brain shows less activity in the amygdala and hippocampus, which deal with fear and anxiety, so that she can relax and enjoy her orgasm. Her orgasm generally lasts longer than his by at least 10 seconds and scientific imaging reveals that female orgasm fires in 80 regions of the brain!

During intercourse, increased amounts of adrenaline are released from the adrenal glands. This chemical amplifies the circulatory system with each heart contraction.

Phase 5 – Resolution
After orgasm, the body goes back to its normal pre-arousal state; muscles relax, the penis becomes soft and the testicles descend back down to their usual place. Heartbeat and breathing slows down and lots of men feel so relaxed that they just want to go to sleep. After orgasm, men release a cocktail of chemicals including prolactin, a hormone that is linked to feelings of sexual satisfaction, hence the smile on his face. He also releases a burst of oxytocin causing him to feel sleepy.

Cooling down for women is defined by how long it takes to get her pulse rate back down to normal and for the rush of blood from her pelvis to subside. Blood pressure and pulse gradually return to pre-arousal levels. Swelling in the genitals and other areas decreases. The labia minora return to their normal color. The clitoris re-emerges from under the clitoral hood and returns to its normal size within about ten minutes. Muscles relax and organs and tissues resume their original positions.

It's important for a woman to cuddle after sex as it releases oxytocin and makes her feel more intimate towards her partner. For men, the benefit of cuddling can lead to increased sexual satisfaction, so fall asleep if you must as long as it's with your arms wrapped around each other.

Oh My, The Big O

For something so juicy, the formal definition of "orgasm" is quite dry. Webster's Dictionary defines orgasm as "Intense or paroxysmal excitement; *especially*: an explosive discharge of neuromuscular tensions at the height of sexual arousal that is usually accompanied by the ejaculation of semen in the male and by vaginal contractions in the female." This basically means a sudden burst of energy, which allows your body to release tension. At the point of orgasm, or climax, a euphoric energy is released throughout the body and causes a strong tightening of most muscles in the body, which basically means ... yes, please.

- ♥ Orgasm enables us to surrender complete control.

- ♥ Orgasm is the best form of escape from reality.

- ♥ Orgasm is the most natural high.

- ♥ Orgasm is wired to our brain, not between our legs.

- ♥ Orgasm gives us indisputable confidence.

- ♥ Orgasm teaches us to accept who we are.

- ♥ Orgasm satisfies us physically.

- ♥ Orgasm satisfies us emotionally.

- ♥ Orgasm can be a spiritual experience.

- ♥ Orgasm can be addictive.

- ♥ Orgasm should not be hurried or pushed by anyone.

- ♥ Orgasm can unite two partners into one.

In both sexes, an area in the frontal lobes of the brain, called the lateral orbitofrontal cortex (OFC), shuts down during orgasm. This region is used for decision-making, obviously not a primary function when reaching an orgasm.

The brain's pleasure center, made up of the amygdala, nucleus accumbens, ventral tegmental area, cerebellum and pituitary gland, is ignited during sexual activity. Also known as the reward circuit, this part of the brain processes all kinds of pleasures, including sex, laughter, and certain kinds of drug use. When this section of the brain was scanned during sexual activity, scientists at the University of Groningen in the Netherlands discovered that there was little difference in the brain patterns of men and women during orgasm. They also discovered something else: an orgasm makes you lose control. Researcher Janniko R. Georgiadis states, "It's the seat of reason and behavioral control. But when you have an orgasm, you lose control" and Dr. Gert Holstege has been quoted as saying that there is little difference between a brain during orgasm and a brain on heroin. "95% is the same."

Sex is our second basic instinct after self-preservation because it leads to the continuation of our species. Not that you need any convincing that orgasms feel good, but did you know that they are also healthy? Several studies have hypothesized that hormones released during arousal and orgasm, specifically oxytocin and DHEA, an endogenous hormone that serves as precursor to male and female sex hormones, may also have protective effects against cancer and heart disease.

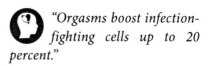

"Orgasms boost infection-fighting cells up to 20 percent."

– Dr. Daniel G. Amen

NEURO-CISE: ORGASM, DUO

Euphoric, mind-blowing, earth shattering, energy-melting orgasms are also a natural way to forget about all of our daily hassles and pain, so why wouldn't we want to feel like we are on top of the world?

The Key to Female Orgasm

The word "clitoris" is derived from the ancient Greek word for "key", hence the key to female sexuality and orgasm or simplistically, the female version of the penis. It is also very similar to the penis with erectile tissue that grows in size when stimulated, but unlike the penis, the clitoris can't pee or ejaculate and only has one function: sexual pleasure.

Oral Delights for Her

Many women are able to orgasm by oral clitoral stimulation alone in just a few minutes while other women may need a half-hour or so.

Getting into various oral sex positions is an added enjoyment. Especially when she is the center of attention. Encourage your partner to lie back comfortably with a pillow under her head and another under her buttocks. Raising her pelvis with a pillow will provide you with the best access to her clitoris. It will also help alleviate strain from your neck. Explore her vulva, the entire outside of the vagina with circular tongue motions and make a conscious effort to maintain eye contact with her as it increases the intimacy between the two of you.

Get her mons (pubic hair area) as wet as you can with your mouth and passionately make out with it. When it comes to oral sex, enthusiasm is even more important than technique. Use your hands to draw her hips and pelvis into your face.

Using your tongue as your utensil, French kiss the vulva and lips of the vagina, paying special attention to the clitoris. Kissing the vagina demands lots of tongue so use the flat of your tongue with consistent long strokes, pressure and speed from the bottom to the top of her vaginal opening. A good kissing tip is to kiss her vagina the same way as you kiss her mouth.

Gently lick with a pointy tongue around the clitoral hood, and then on top, before pulling the hood back, as some women's clitoral nerve endings are more sensitive than others. Then lick her clitoris from side to side like a windshield wiper or wrap your lips around the clitoris, and start sucking lightly, then add more pressure until she signals you to stop.

Make humming sounds with your lips so they vibrate on her clitoris because mmmmmm is not just a sound, it's a sensation that can awaken her most erotic senses. She won't need a vibrator! Then follow up with some very light finger taps directly on the clitoris for sexual peak sensations and go back and forth with your mouth and your finger until it takes her over the edge.

A study in The Journal of Sexual Medicine shows that the clitoris becomes 15 to 20 percent larger on the 14th day of a woman's menstrual cycle, thanks to the extra blood flow, making the spot even more sensitive.

"G" is for Good

Statistics show that 78% of women do not explore the inside of their own bodies, yet the Grafenberg spot (The G spot) - located just 2 inches inside the opening to the vagina - can bring about longer, deeper, more powerful orgasms than a clitoral orgasm. Located on the anterior or front wall of the vagina, between the opening and the cervix, this area is often found to be extremely sensitive to stimulation.

Begin by inserting one or two fingers and discover her G-spot while licking her clitoris, but make sure that she is already wet and willing. Begin by resting your thumb on her clitoris while inserting the middle finger of your prominent hand in a "come here" motion into her vagina, palm up. Just imagine there is a clock on the inside of the vagina and you are stroking from 6 o'clock (at the bottom of her vaginal opening) to 12 o'clock (her G-spot). Use long strokes, creating an energetic circuit between your thumb and finger. Now replace your thumb on her clitoris with your mouth and tap her G-spot with your finger while you lick her clitoris. If all goes well, she will have an internal and external orgasm at the same time and you'll be a hero.

Let her push you away when her orgasm has ended. A woman's orgasm can last much longer than a man's, especially a clitoral and G-spot orgasm combined, which can result in deeper more intense spasms, followed by waves of pleasure that make her feel like she is floating on a cloud.

Afterwards, she may still be very sensitive to touch, so just cup your hand over her vagina gently and hold her. This is a very romantic gesture, which actually holds sexual energy inside her for as long as possible.

The G-spot can also be reached using a specially designed vibrator that has a curved tip.

Research by Dr. Beverly Whipple, author of *The G Spot and Other Recent Discoveries About Human Sexuality* validated women who experienced G-spot orgasms and who ejaculated.

Female ejaculation has been documented in ancient Asia for many thousands of years. Here in the Western world scientists are finally accepting it as a reality and women of all ages are enjoying the experience of ejaculating during orgasm. I believe that every woman can ejaculate if she is stimulated correctly and if she knows how to control her Kegel muscles. It's estimated that less than 10% of women ejaculate, or at least admit to it. Some women who experience ejaculation admit that the feeling is like an intense orgasmic release, much stronger and longer than a clitoral orgasm. Female ejaculation can be attained with stimulation of the G-spot, but the bladder should be emptied first so that the ejaculation doesn't have much urine in it. The ejaculate fluid is protein based, much like semen, but it's thinner and of course it doesn't have any sperm. In summary, female ejaculation is a normal natural occurrence, so why not try it? You might like it!

Oral Pleasure for Him

Most men will confess that erotic stimulation is about 70% visual and 30% physical, which is why many men love to watch their partner lavish them with oral pleasure. The most sensitive area of the penis is the small strip of skin that joins the head of the penis to the foreskin, also known as the "Sweet Spot" and clinically known as the "Frenulum." This area has lots of sensitive nerve endings and extra oral stimulation will make your man very happy. You can use your hands in addition to your mouth and place one on his shaft with the other around his testes as you massage them gently.

Speaking of testes, the scrotum is the skin that encompasses them and every man's testes are part of his penis, but many men complain that they are often neglected. It's your job to find out if he enjoys having his testes caressed, licked or sucked. Be gentle as they are sensitive and be aware that prior to ejaculation, the scrotum will become firmer and rise up towards the penis.

Wrap your lips tightly around his glans, the (head) of the penis, and use plenty of suction by using your mouth as a vacuum to simulate a popping sound. I call this the head-popper, which can be very erotic for men to watch, feel and hear. For some men, the foreskin covers the glans when they are flaccid, while other men have had their foreskin removed, however, when a man is erect it pulls back. For men with lots of foreskin, suck his foreskin between your lips and use your tongue to circle in between the foreskin glans. This is often referred to as "tongue docking."

His Million Dollar Point

The man has his very own good spot, also known as the prostate, which can be accessed internally or externally. There is an ancient Taoist technique called the "Million Dollar Point" that stimulates the Prostate without going inside the anus. Start by slowly sliding your fingers up and down the perineum (the landing strip between his anus to his testicles). Feel for a small indentation the size of a pea, about midway, and gently press inward with your two fingers. Many men are able to feel their prostate gland through this point, so it can result in an earth-shattering, mind-blowing orgasm for him.

Internal prostate massage may arouse you or your male partner to new levels of intimate pleasure because the area of the anus is surrounded with sensitive nerve endings. Before doing prostate massage, you should have a latex glove or finger cots ready, and you'll certainly want plenty of lubricant. I call the prostate his "Hero Spot" because it takes a hero to be adventurous, secure in his masculinity and trusting with his partner in order to embark on Hero Spot exploration.

The prostate is the size of a walnut located about 4 cm inside the anus and can be effectively stimulated by the insertion of a finger or vibrator. A comfortable position is for the man to lie on his back with his knees raised and be sure that he is aroused, ready and willing to proceed.

- ♥ Lubricate your finger cover, and rub the outside of the anus before inserting it palm up, in a "come hither" motion slowly.

- ♥ As his sphincter muscles contract, wait until he is ready for you to go deeper.

- ♥ Push your finger inside and apply a light pressure either tapping or stroking towards his perineum. Ask your partner what feels best. Some men say their pleasure zone is just one knuckle inside the anus; others are deeper and enjoy more vigorous thrusting.

- ♥ Ask him to share his feelings of pleasure, anticipation and concern and if he would like to try it again.

- ♥ The prostate can also be reached using specially designed stimulators that have curved and contoured tips with grip handles to make insertion and removal safe and easy.

Choose Your Orgasm

There are many different kinds of orgasm that you can experience from stimulation of different parts of your body. Each one will create its own feelings ranging from quick, short, localized, deep, concentrated, to full body orgasms. This is your opportunity to experiment with as many different kinds of orgasm as you can. Remember that orgasm is good for your health so it's doctor's orders!

A UniGasm

This is an orgasm where stimulation is directed to one primary erogenous zone such as the penis, prostate, testicles, clitoris, G-spot, anus, or nipples. Nipple stimulation for men and women can produce an orgasm, though it's not as common as some of the other erogenous zones.

NippleGasm

According to scientists at Rutgers University, brain scans show that when women stroke their nipples, it activates the same area of the brain as clitoral and vaginal stimulations.

For women, having their breasts caressed and nipples sucked releases oxytocin, the chemical that makes them feel like they are in love. Masters and Johnson discovered that one percent of women were able to achieve orgasm from breast stimulation alone. This is an area that many men enjoy stimulating during foreplay, but rarely think of as having orgasmic potential.

To give memorable oral sex on her breasts and nipples you need to understand that the size of her breasts have nothing to do with the sensitivity. Ask her if she gets turned on by having her breasts played with. If so, then follow these directions:

1. Begin by caressing and licking both of her breasts, and not just her nipples.

2. Alternate each one as you use the flat of your tongue in lapping motions all around her breasts covering every centimeter. Follow your tongue with light fingertip caresses, leaving her nipples until last.

3. When both breasts are suitably wet from your tongue, cup

your hand over one breast at a time so that the tip of her nipple rests in between your thumb and your index finger. Squeeze the fingers together so that you raise her nipple slightly, and then begin licking it with the tip of your tongue in circular motions.

4. After about a dozen licks or so, pucker your lips around the nipple and suck gently but firmly; let your head bob up and down simultaneously.

5. To enhance oral nipple sensation, put an ice cube in your mouth while lavishing her orally.

6. Don't forget to give equal attention to both breasts and nipples. When she is climaxing do not stop or change what you are doing. Let her push you away when she is ready.

For male nipple stimulation, the directions are pretty much the same, except men are usually more interested in having immediate nipple contact with deeper vacuum sucking motions, not so much teasing around the nipple area. Some men enjoy having their nipples nibbled on. It's up to you to find out how much pain or pleasure your man wants on his nipples. Some people have one nipple that is more sensitive than the other. While you suck on one, you can pinch the other one and then ask him which one feels most erotic. You could be the first one to introduce him to a UniGasm through his nipples. Now that's what I call creating a lasting mammary (I mean memory)!

A BiGasm

Many people are experienced with various forms of dual stimulation—a penis and a tongue, a vagina and a tongue, a finger and a tongue, and various other combinations. This will be more intense than a UniGasm, so it's worth exploring. Here are some ideal ways to create two points of stimulation at the same time:

♥ Licking his testicles while masturbating his penis

♥ Sucking on her clitoris while stimulating her G-spot.

♥ Sucking his penis while stimulating his prostate.

♥ Licking her perineum while fingering her vagina

Have fun experimenting with different combinations on your partner's body. Ask for feedback so that you know which combinations are most exciting for you both.

The Blended Orgasm

A blended orgasm is much like the BiGasm with a little twist. The intention for the blended orgasm is to make it last much longer by teasing your partner and stimulating one primary erogenous zone, then teasing another, then going back to the first and so on.

1. Start by choosing your favorite orgasm technique (such as oral stimulation on the clitoris for a woman and oral stimulation on the penis for a guy).

2. Get aroused to a level 6 on your pleasure scale, and then switch to another orgasm technique you enjoy (such as G-spot for a woman and prostate for a guy) and get aroused to a level 7 this time.

3. Switch back to the first technique, raise your arousal level to 8 and then back to the second technique at least three times before reaching a level 10 on your orgasm scale.

This orgasm technique is a wonderful way to monitor your pleasure scale and is most beneficial for men who suffer from premature ejaculation. Whenever they feel like they are about to reach their orgasm, they move their attention to another erogenous zone to distract from reaching the point of no return too soon.

The TriGasm for Her

So, here's the revolution, the ultimate orgasm, the TriGasm. A female TriGasm is the result of arousing three points of pleasure, the clitoris, G-spot, and anus simultaneously. Here are some tips for you and your partner as you go off on your TriGasm exploration.

1. The woman should lie back while her partner lavishes her clitoris with oral pleasure until she has reached a level 8 on a pleasure scale of 1 to 10.

2. Change course and stimulate her vulva (outside of the vagina) in small circles with your tongue for 2 minutes.

3. Return to the clitoris and orally increase her level of pleasure to a 9, almost to the point of no return.

4. At this peak, insert your forefinger palm up into her vagina and find her G-spot, then tap, tap, tap it gently towards her navel.

5. Simultaneously with step four, stimulate her anus gently with a feather, a pinky or a vibrator to bring her to a huge, extraordinary TriGasm!

The TriGasm for Him

The TriGasm for men is also the result of stimulating three points of pleasure, the penis, the testicles and the anus simultaneously.

1. The man should lie back while his partner lavishes the head of his penis with some good oral suction until he reaches a level 8 on a pleasure scale of 1 to 10.

2. Then use your mouth and tongue to stimulate his testicles for 2 minutes while you masturbate his penis with your hand.

3. Return to the penis orally and increase his level of pleasure to a 9, almost to the point of no return.

4. At this peak, fondle his testicles as you continue to orally

delight his penis and insert your forefinger palm up into his anus to find his prostate gland, then tap, tap, tap it gently.

5. If all goes well, he'll have an unforgettable, enormous TriGasm!

The BrainGasm

The BrainGasm concept is to slowly build the mental and emotional intensity between partners. Sex starts between the ears as your brain influences the kind of sex you want to have - romantic, playful, sensual, intimate, erotic or wild. By concentrating on the interconnection you share on the deepest level, a firecracker turns into a full sky of explosive fireworks.

1. With millions of nerve endings in the brain devoted to the lips, passionate kissing is essential to achieving a BrainGasm. During a long wet make-out kiss, adrenaline makes your heart race while the nucleus accumbens controls the release of dopamine (a craving signal) from the reward center of your brain.

2. Once the juices are flowing, focus on your partner with your full attention by looking deep into their eyes to release oxytocin, the bonding chemical that increases desire and establishes a greater sense of intimacy.

3. Put your prominent hand on each other's heart to light the emotional fire centers for a heart-mind-body connection. The amygdala induces sexual energy from the brain as balanced serotonin levels make you feel intense pleasure emotions, as if two hearts beat as one.

4. Whisper into your partner's ear how you are going to sexually satisfy them, and take in their scent of arousal. Smell is the most primitive of all of our senses that comes from the olfactory bulb, part of the brain's limbic system, an area so closely connected with memory and emotion it's often called the "Emotional Brain."

5. Take your partner's breath away by using your breath around their most sensitive erogenous zones from the top of their neck to the tip of their toes. When you blow your cool breath on the left side of your partner's body, you are stimulating the right side of their brain. Watch your partner's muscles contract with pleasure, controlled by the cerebellum.

6. Your partner should be begging you to touch them by now and with the first erotic touch on the nipples, toes or sexual organs, the brains sensory cortex region fires up. Neurons that are linked to your various erogenous zones communicate with the sensory cortex, to eventually activate the brain regions that produce orgasm. You may be interested to know that the toes are located next to the clitoris in the sensory cortex of the female brain.

7. Make love to activate the hippocampus, a region of the brain that evokes mind-blowing sensations, while the frontal cortex induces erotic fantasies and the cerebellum triggers body-melting sexual tension – this can all result in an earth shattering, energy melting, all-embracing BrainGasm.

NEURO-CISE: HANDS-FREE ORGASM, SOLO

Since the brain is the most erotic organ in the body, it should be no surprise that you can think your way to orgasm. Sexual thoughts can activate the brain just like sexual touching does. If you've ever enjoyed looking at porn, you'll know what I'm talking about. Visuals of people having sex can automatically trigger your body into a state of arousal, making women wet and giving men erections. If you continued to watch erotica without touching yourself, you could still experience a full-blown orgasm. Even if you're not into porn, you can achieve a mind over body orgasm by tapping into all of your five senses.

Sexologist and Professor Emerita at Rutgers University Dr. Beverly Whipple is often referred to as "the inventor of the G-spot" based on a book she co-authored in 1982 entitled *The G-Spot and Other*

Recent Discoveries About Human Sexuality. Through her work, Mr. Whipple has documented that some women can achieve orgasm from visual stimulation alone, without touch. She states, "The point is that women can experience orgasms and sexual pleasure from many forms of stimuli. It does not have to be through genital stimulation."

To begin your hands-free orgasm, use only your imagination to think about what your partner's tongue would feel like between your legs and what he or she smells like when fully aroused. Visualize what they look like naked. Imagine touching, kissing, licking and tasting his or her body. Hear them moaning with pleasure. Become aware of your own feelings as you let your excitement build. The trick here is not to touch yourself, but to let the ebb and flow of your orgasm take you on a mental journey to sexual ecstasy. This can also be fun to do with a partner as a safe sex activity.

Love Is Work

Life is full of enough challenges outside the bedroom so why not do what is necessary to keep things safe and warm within the bedroom? Besides, since we're talking about intimacy and sexuality, the research is so much more fun than any day job. I mean, if you have to decide between spreadsheets and spread legs, where would you rather put your focus for a few hours?

There's no denying that it takes a lot of work to sustain a healthy, passionate relationship, but the work is worth it. One way to add some fun and excitement to this process is to make it a full sensory exploration. By understanding and incorporating all of the senses, it becomes even easier to enhance the intimate connection. Read on as we explore the concept of Sensory Connection.

CHAPTER FOUR
Sensory Connection

The full human experience is a complicated dance between the outside world and our internal processing system. And in this dance, our senses are the music. What we see, touch, taste, hear, and feel and our emotional reaction to those things influences our every move, aided by the mysterious "sixth sense" of intuition.

This music of life is created by the orchestra of sensory receptors that detect and respond to various stimuli, such as light, sound, motion, pressure, and temperature.

"Love is the poetry of the senses."

– Honoré de Balzac

These neurons hum the melodies that enrich our senses with the most basic tools for survival. As these signals send messages to the brain, several key areas are triggered, including:

♥ Amygdala, the emotions manager

♥ Nucleus accumbens, the dopamine controller

- ♥ Ventral tegmental area (VTA), the dopamine releaser

- ♥ Cerebellum, the muscle function regulator

- ♥ Pituitary gland, the distributor of beta-endorphins (which decrease pain), oxytocin (which increases feelings of trust) and vasopressin (the bonding hormone)

All of these instruments work together to send messages to our mind and body. I see my partner undress and I get aroused. I smell fresh flowers and I think of a first date. I taste chocolate and I remember a special Valentine's Day. I touch silk sheets and it reminds me of a hotel getaway. I hear my partner moan and I want to move closer. I know my partner is going to call in the moment before the phone rings.

By understanding how these particular sensory songs are sung, we are able to create the playlist for a truly enriched relationship. Let's take a closer look at the instruments that come together to form the soundtrack to our lives.

Sensory Attraction

To connect with a new person you are attracted to, we know that eye contact is the most potent trigger, as it activates the brain's reward center and releases oxytocin, the feel-good chemical that's discharged when you feel bonded with someone physically or emotionally.

To get a new person hooked on you, you need to trigger desire and create memorable dates that will release addictive forming chemicals such as dopamine and noradrenaline. Since the most powerful of all of our senses is smell, you can activate intense feelings by wearing a brand of perfume or cologne that your intended new partner loves, or surround them with the aroma of familiar foods, which is especially potent for men.

> "When he experiences something that he associates with falling in love with you, those intense, sensual memories trigger a positive physical reaction and generate instant longing."
>
> - Jeffrey Bernstein, PhD

You've Got The Magic Touch

If I had to describe touch as a musical style, I would say it's the dance music of our lives. It's the rhythm, the pounding, and the desire to be close enough to physically feel a connection. It's an embrace, a kiss, two heartbeats close enough together that they pulse as one.

There is no denying the importance of human touch. Our other senses develop after birth, but the sense of touch develops while still in the womb and remains highly important throughout life. In fact, it could be considered the most important sense. Throughout the body, inside and out, nerve endings send messages to the brain regarding four kinds of touch sensations: cold, heat, pressure, and pain, including any physical warnings that may be life threatening.

Different from all the other senses, the sense of touch involves our bodies from head to toe. That's because the sensory receptors that allow us to feel things are located in our skin, though some parts of our skin have many more receptors than others. According to an article from *Johns Hopkins Magazine,* our fingertips have about 3,000 touch receptors each. The trunks of our bodies have about the same amount of receptors as just one fingertip.

Positive touch may also be associated with overall wellbeing. The Touch Research Institute at the University of Miami performed a study of ten infants (starting at ten weeks old), whose mothers were taught to stroke their infant's backs. At six months of age, these babies had fewer colds, sniffles, vomiting and diarrhea than infants in the control group, whose mothers had not been taught to stroke their infants.

What about as we grow older? Even though we have noticeable loss in nerve fiber and decreased acuity in the sense of touch over the years, it appears our needs for tactile stimulation may actually increase. One has only to observe the responses of older people to a caress, an embrace, a pat on the hand or clasp, to appreciate how vitally necessary such experiences are for their wellbeing. Scientific evidence shows the course and outcome of many an illness has been greatly influenced by the quality of tactile support the individual has received before and during the illness.

Aline Newton, developer of the Physical Intelligence Program at MIT, states that touch impacts our thinking, feeling, sensory and motor systems. It also has been shown to have a positive emotional impact and appears to affect multiple brain regions at conscious and unconscious levels. The brain's map of the body is held in the homunculus, located on the surface of the brain. With the sense of touch, receptors in the skin and muscles transmit signals via the spinal cord and medulla to this area of the brain, firing up the neurons. This body map is 'plastic', meaning it is not fixed, but rather can change based on experience and learning.

"Physical touch is one of love's strongest voices."

– Dr. Gary Chapman

There are two types of brain plasticity. The first is *Functional Plasticity*, which refers to the brain's capacity to move functions from a damaged area of the brain to other undamaged areas of the brain. The second type of brain plasticity is known as *Structural Plasticity*, which refers to the brain's capability to change its physical structure as a result of learning. This learning, however, is not as simple as just exploring a new sexual position. It must be the extended education of something that takes time, with new information such as a new language, a new hobby, even a new lifestyle. Becoming a massage therapist, or practicing Tantra or BDSM (bondage, domination/discipline, Sadism and Masochism) can change the physical structure of the brain.

It is also possible to heighten the power of touch through concentration. In many instances, touch is overlooked as part of our multi-tasking life. For example, if you hold hands with your partner at a movie, you are receiving the messages of touch, but the larger portion of your brain's focus is on the visuals and sounds of the film, as well as the taste of your hot popcorn. But if later at home, you lay in bed next to each other in the dark and take each other's hand, the sensation is much more pronounced because your interlocked fingers now have your full attention.

NEURO-CISE: SENSORY, DUO

It's important to learn how your partner likes to be touched and share where you like to be touched. Some simple ways to incorporate more physical contact in your relationship include:

- ♥ Hug more often, making sure each hug lasts at least six seconds in order to release the "cuddle hormone" oxytocin.

- ♥ A head massage is not only relaxing but also releases oxytocin.

- ♥ Take the time to explore each other's bodies using your fingertips without the intent of sexual release.

- ♥ Communicate love with your facial expressions, hand motions and body language as much as your voice.

- ♥ If a man is involved in your intimate activities, kiss for at least 10 seconds in order to release testosterone from the man's mouth.

NEURO-CISE: EROGENOUS ZONE, DUO

Becoming aware of erogenous zones is a great way to enhance physical relationships. These "pleasure points" produce erotic feelings when stimulated.

Before embarking on the pleasure journey with a partner, it's a great idea to experience some of your own personal erogenous zones. You can discover your own sexuality by looking at yourself in the mirror, then touching yourself to find out what really feels good to you. Take the time to do this. You're the one who will receive the reward. Get to know your entire body from head to

"It is our brain chemicals that govern how we can successfully interact with one another."

– Dr. John Gray

toe, outside and inside, and discover your own erogenous zones so that you can communicate your turn-ons to your partner.

One often-overlooked area that can boost arousal and even magnify orgasmic intensity is the ear. This is a wonderful place to start in exploring your partner's erogenous zones.

Along the outer edge of the ear is a C-shaped pleasure zone that responds to finger caressing, warm or cool breath, kissing, licking, sucking and delicate biting. Don't rush, take your time and be gentle as you tease your partner by moving your tongue and lips gently around the C-spot. Just the right kind of stimulation can be so seductive that it sends erotic chills through the body and creates sexual anticipation of what's to come.

The C-spot has infinite nerve endings and more than 120 acupressure points that correspond to various parts of the body, including the genital region. For some people it is the highest sensitivity in their bodies that can result in an "eargasm" during foreplay or while making love.

When you're ready to explore your partner more thoroughly, have them get naked and lay back for you on the bed. Ask them to close their eyes and count to ten to get relaxed. Then, very slowly let them feel your breath against their skin without touching it. When they are not expecting it, lightly brush your fingertips over their body, carefully caressing each area a half inch at a time from head to toe. Have them rate the sensations from 1 to

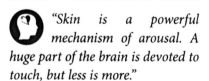 *"Skin is a powerful mechanism of arousal. A huge part of the brain is devoted to touch, but less is more."*

– Dr. Helen Fisher

10. (This score is about their sensitivity to touch and not a rating of your performance). Explore both the front and back. It is your job to memorize the areas your partner rates higher than a seven so that you can revisit them later during a more intense sexual experience.

Once you know your partner's hot zones, you can explore them even further with a variety of accouterments, ranging from mild to wild. Consider adding some of the following pleasure enhancers to your adult toy box.

- ♥ **Feathers:** boas, fans, ostrich, peacock, duster, plume

- ♥ **Vibrators:** silicone, plastic, glass, jelly, latex, cyberskin, chrome

- ♥ **Lubricants:** warming, cooling, numbing, tingling, flavored, silicone, oil-based, water-based, organic

- ♥ **Scarves:** silk, satin, various furs, velvet, cashmere, leather, lace, chiffon

- ♥ **Whips & Paddles:** leather, horse hair, rubber, mops, rabbit fur, flat braids, wood, sheepskin

- ♥ **Beads:** Crystal, shell, wood, pearl, clay, Mardi Gras beads, gemstones

- ♥ **Lingerie:** Charmeuse, satin, lycra, spandex, cotton, lace, sheer nylon, silk, PVC, leather

- ♥ Breath, hair, fingernails, tongue, mouth, water, ice, bubble bath, Jacuzzi and anything else that you and your partner can imagine, as long as it feel good for both of you.

In Your Eyes

There's an incredibly visceral connection between touch and sight. When we see something we like, we are drawn to feel it. I compare vision to pop music. It's colorful, bright, emotional, and universal. Humans are highly visual animals and there's nothing quite like the feelings generated by the things we see. What can compare to a glorious sunset, the extraordinary sight of a long lost friend, or the first time you see your new lover smile?

And who isn't familiar with the phrase "love at first sight"? This romantic concept has inspired countless songs, poems, movies and embarrassing text messages and Facebook posts. The phenomenon may actually have a basis in science. The findings of several studies have shown that more men have proven to believe in the concept of love at first sight than women. This is largely because men respond to physical attributes more quickly than women and women also take longer to settle into a feeling of trust.

Considered to be the most complex sense, vision is an intricate process of data being transferred from the optical nerves to the various parts of the brain responsible for naming things, remembering faces and places, and the emotional reactions to what is being seen. The brain combines the messages from both eyes in order to create a single three-dimensional image. To complicate things further, the image received on the retina is upside down due to the focusing action of the lens and the brain has to flip the image to provide the right-side-up view.

Sight is such an integral part of the human experience that nearly 50% of the brain's sensory resources are dedicated to vision, according to Dr. John Medina, developmental molecular biologist and best-selling author of *Brain Rules*. That means that vision alone uses as much of the brain as all the other senses combined.

In a relationship, it's important to make a concerted effort to not just look, but to see. This is especially important for those in long-term relationships. The longer we spend with people,

 "It's not what you look at that matters, it's what you see."

– Henry David Thoreau

the more easily we forget to pay attention to the details. It is quite possible to become unaware of something one sees every day. That's one of the great capacities of the brain.

Can you easily move through your home in the dark because you know where everything is without needing to constantly see it? The same thing can happen with the people around us. We forget to look at them because we know what they look like but, in reality, the image we have in our head is purely a memory unless we take the time to fully focus and look. This phenomenon explains why a haircut, weight loss, or a new shirt might be missed. Even though we are side by side, unless we turn to really look, the person we see in our peripheral vision is only the "photograph" we have from the last time we paid attention.

NEURO-CISE: VISUAL, DUO

Romance and love are richly enhanced by the sense of sight. If you invest time, energy and focus into the visual aspects of your relationship, you will absolutely create a stronger bond. Some easy ways to do this include:

- ♥ Send your partner an email or text message photo of your smiling face.

- ♥ Wear a small surprise that you can secretly reveal in public, like a temporary tattoo of your partner's nickname. It doesn't have to be naughty, just meaningful.

- ♥ Undress for your partner, slowly and seductively.

- ♥ Make love with a commitment to eye contact.

- ♥ Dim the lights or use colored fabric to drape over lampshades, candles, wear lingerie or pose in front of a mirror, tidy up your place, pretend a VIP is coming to visit, turn your bedroom into a romantic boudoir.

The importance of vision in romantic connection helps explain the popularity of romantic movies. Do you have a favorite movie that you turn to when you need to feel "'in the mood" or one that reminds you of the romance in the world when you're having a blue day?

Get into character and reenact your favorite love scenes from movies. A few notable films to check out for this are: *Body Heat, A Walk On the*

Moon, Before Sunset, Bull Durham, Shortbus, The Pornographer, Intimacy, Brokeback Mountain, 9 1/2 Weeks, and *In the Realm of the Senses.*

Reenact your favorite kissing scenes from movies with your partner. Whether it's from *Pirates of the Caribbean, Closer, Twilight, The Notebook, Mulholland Drive,* or *A Single Man,* this could be the perfect way to create a kissing sensation that surpasses your expectations.

Pretend that you are the writer, director, and star of a hot steamy movie and your partner is your co-star. Give him or her a kissing scene to perform on you.

Hollywood may give us false hope for "happily ever after" but it also reminds us that love is a complicated, funny, challenging, scary, exciting adventure. Are you living the kind of the love that could ignite the silver screen?

Seeing What The Body Says

If you've heard that 55% of communication is based on non-verbal body language, 38% is all about the tone of voice and only 7% is based on actual words spoken, then you are familiar with researcher Professor Albert Mehrabian whose findings are quoted worldwide, and have become known as the 7%-38%-55% rule. So it's incredibly important to remain aware of eye contact, facial expressions and posture, especially during intimate discussions.

Speaking of eye contact, according to Joe Riggs, acclaimed mentalist, hypnotherapist and author, it's actually possible to watch a person's eyes alone as an indication of whether or not they are telling the truth. "When asking someone a direct question, a left or right eye movement can mean the difference between the truth and a lie. Looking to the left indicates a made up answer as their eyes are showing a constructed image or sound whereas looking to the right would indicate a "remembered" voice or image, and thus would be the truth. Remember that every person is different so never base a conclusion on just one observation."

Have you ever paid attention to the body language of other people when you have an opportunity for observation? The next time you are in a restaurant, a park or other social environment, take a moment to look at how other people are interacting. Without hearing any words, how much information can you decipher? The man with his arms crossed while his female companion speaks - is he disinterested or is he angry? The girl leaning forward with a smile as she orders coffee from the boy looking away - is she flirting and, if so, is he interested?

If you'd like to improve the way you use body language in your own life, mentally, physically and emotionally, you can simply be aware of your posture by standing up straight and boldly putting your hands on your hips in order for your brain to increase 20% testosterone and decrease 25% cortisol, according to a study by social psychologist Amy Cuddy at Harvard.

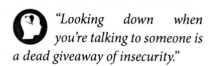 *"Looking down when you're talking to someone is a dead giveaway of insecurity."*

- Sharon Sayler

NEURO-CISE: VISUAL, SOLO

- ♥ A smile is an open door of approval and if you keep a consistent gaze with the person you are talking to at the same time, you've got a sensory visual connection.

- ♥ Relax your shoulders and have your palms facing upwards with your fingers facing the person you are talking to, as open hand gestures signify that you are open to exchanging ideas with them.

- ♥ Point your feet towards the person you are interested in and see if their feet are pointed towards you, which is a good sign and means they want you to approach them.

- ♥ Lean in to conversations and nod when you agree with something being said, so that you both feel like you are on the same page.

♥ Don't hold anything in front of your chest. Covering your heart creates a guarded perception.

♥ As a couple, when you both mimic each other's moves on the dance floor or order the same drinks, you clearly are in sync mentally, physically and emotionally.

The bottom line is that if you're not feeling confident, then fake it until you make it and turn your happy button on, as your brain won't know the difference between what is real and what is imagined.

The Sound Of Your Voice

If the sight of something can light a fire within us, than the sound of it has the power to warm our soul. In our musical catalog of senses, I classify hearing as the classical repertoire. There's no denying the seductive power of sound. A whisper. A groan. A love song. Hearing your name followed by the words "I love you." Sound is like an inner massage; cells in your body respond to vibrations and release energy. Music, laughter and words have power to heal and arouse.

As the auditory cortex receives sound messages with the frontal and parietal lobes, the brain identifies these and defines the direction and distance of these sounds by merging information

 "Sound is the vocabulary of nature."

– Pierre Schaeffer

received from both ears. It's a highly complicated exchange of information involving intricate instruments. The malleus, incus and stapes (otherwise known as the hammer, anvil and stirrup) are the smallest bones in the human body and are full size at birth. All three together could fit on a penny.

Using sound in healing has been gaining momentum in the medical industry. "I believe that sound can play a role in virtually any medical disorder, since it redresses imbalances on every level of physiologic functioning," writes Dr. Mitchell Gaynor in his book *The Healing Power of Sound: Recovery from Life-Threatening Illness Using Sound, Voice and Music*. Furthermore, Dr. Gaynor sees sound beginning to play a large part in the trend of mindful medicine, where the whole person is treated, not just the part that is injured.

Just as physical ailments can be caused by emotional distress, our bodies respond to positive emotions with better health, which can be brought about with sound-based therapy that shapes and shifts our mood.

For instance, if you're sitting in a park on a quiet day, how is your mood affected by the sudden chirping of birds or children laughing nearby versus the explosive blare of a car alarm going off? Or consider the various sounds in your local gym. Compare the differences in music between an intense aerobics class and a meditative yoga class. Whether our conscious mind is aware of it or not, our bodies take cues, emotional and otherwise, from these auditory messages.

Speaking of music, this incredible art form is strongly associated with the brain's reward system. According to Robert Zatorre, professor of neurology and neurosurgery at the Montreal Neurological Institute, this reward system is that part of the brain that gives value to things and lets us know if they are important for survival. Music also releases the pleasure chemical dopamine in the brain and imaging has revealed that this is similar to how the brain responds to food and sex. "I think there's enough evidence to say that musical experience, musical exposure, musical training, all of those things change your brain," says Dr. Charles Limb, of Johns Hopkins University. "It allows you to think in a way that you used to not think, and it also trains a lot of other cognitive facilities that have nothing to do with music."

Given the healing and mood-enhancing powers of music, it can be an important element to bring into your love life. Bill Lamb is a music journalist who has been covering the world of pop music since 1999. He says that most of us can think of particular songs we associate with the love relationships of our lives. Many couples bond over a particular song, one that they picked for their wedding dance, or one that was playing during a romantic or exciting adventure. Take the time to revisit your favorite music as a couple and share the happy memories it brings up.

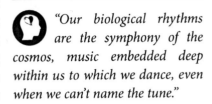

"Our biological rhythms are the symphony of the cosmos, music embedded deep within us to which we dance, even when we can't name the tune."

– Dr. Deepak Chopra

Communicating Love

It's important to pay attention to the sounds of your surroundings, especially as you work to build or rebuild your relationship. Reducing distractions can be hugely beneficial (which is easier said than done if you have kids in the house!). It's also important to become aware of the tone and volume of your own speaking voice. Never underestimate the power of a kind whisper of affection to your partner. Admiration is one of the best compliments you can give someone you care about. It literally means a feeling of pleasure and approval. Telling your partner what a great job they've done or how much you respect and appreciate decisions they've made boosts their self-esteem and opens them up to trusting you with important decisions and events. Your gift keeps on giving as your partner's brain releases the neurochemical oxytocin which wires the brain to seek opportunities to trust and get more of that safe feeling.

NEURO-CISE: SOUND, DUO

One of the most important language adjustments you can make is to use open-ended questions that invite a dialogue instead of a one-word answer. Specific questions can reveal how your partner is feeling. For example, instead of asking, "Weren't you annoyed that the service was so slow at the restaurant?" to which your partner could just say, "Yes," re-phrase to ask, "What did you think about the restaurant, even though the service was so slow?" This will invite a full sentence answer where you can continue the conversation for as long as you want. Here are some more examples:

- ♥ What do you feel about…?

- ♥ What do you think about…?

- ♥ What do you like about…?

- ♥ What do you dislike about…?

- ♥ What do you want to do about…?

- ♥ What might happen if you…?

- ♥ What do you wish would happen if you…?

One couple I counseled had what they described as "relationship-threatening communication issues," and it turned out that the woman rarely allowed her partner space to voice his opinion. Of course he could have offered it up freely, but given the prompts for a "yes" or "no" answer, he always took the bait. Then she would become resentful that he didn't engage in conversation. Simply by incorporating these open-ended questions, their communication issues dissipated.

Compliments are also a great way to show appreciation for your partner because everyone needs to be reminded of all the things that make them lovable. It makes them feel valued. Take some time to do a *Love List* of all the things you love about each other mentally, physically, emotionally, spiritually and sexually. Then take turns reading your list to each other. I use this exercise in my office and love to watch couples react to compliments they haven't heard in years.

Talk Dirty To Me
Lovemaking creates its own form of communication, and one of the best ways to enhance the experience is through erotic talk. Talking Dirty talk is one of the most powerful forms of seduction, and it can make your love life more exciting, more creative, and more fun. It offers a great starting point for other sexual behavior, and has several benefits all on its own:

♥ It helps escape reality

♥ It safely tests sexual boundaries

♥ It increases arousal

♥ It can intensify orgasm

♥ It's fun and naughty

Erotic talk is a great escape from your daily routine, work issues, family problems and other life obstacles that bring you stress. Describe your wants and desires, and guess at theirs, utilizing all the senses you can. Imagine what turns you both on, whether it's a sight, sound, smell, taste, or touch. Keep in mind that, in general, women enjoy implicit fantasies with lots of context and foreplay while men like visually-loaded scenes and explicit action. And remember it's not always about using X-rated words and descriptions. Sometimes the hottest thing to say is a well-placed "yes" against your partner's ear.

If you're intimidated or embarrassed by erotic talk, especially if you've been a shy or silent lover in the past, a great way to begin testing the waters is to read erotic literature to your partner. That way you can get comfortable using naughty words and see what does and doesn't work for you both. It's easier to begin with someone else's words!

NEURO-CISE: SOUND, SOLO

No matter how good your opening line is, it's not going to work if you don't use the proper delivery. Here are some basic rules that will help you to connect with strangers.

♥ Be yourself and don't try to impress by acting like someone else.

♥ Try to make him or her smile or even laugh to get their brain to release feel-good endorphins.

♥ Say his or her name once you find out what it is, as this will give you an immediate advantage, since it grabs the person's full attention.

♥ Use words of a sensory nature such as, "I hear that" or "I can only imagine it" and "I feel the same way."

Make sure to use an appropriate line for the environment you are in. For example, a friendly approach like, "Hi my name is _____, How are you doing today?" can work anywhere from the supermarket to the carwash. A seductive approach, like "You are the sexiest person here tonight" can be effective at a bar or a nightclub, especially if romantic music is playing in the background. A humorous approach might work almost anywhere from a dog park to a bus stop, but not in a hospital where your target date may be visiting someone close to them who is very ill. If you have a dog, one of my favorite lines is "My dog would like to meet your dog, but she/he is very shy." Alternatively, I recommend giving an open-ended compliment such as, "That's a nice bag, where did you get it?" which lets the person know they have a good sense of style and you can then keep the conversation going with positive feedback.

Remember to say something. Anything is better than nothing!

Start by commenting on the other person or the environment, and then sustain the conversation by asking questions and close by getting their phone number.

The Sweet Smell of Success

To me, smell is the country music of the senses. It's the moist air after a rainstorm. It's rose petals on the bed. It's autumn leaves rustling in the wind. Have you ever noticed how quickly a smell can trigger a reaction? I was working with a man once on a creative exercise and when he opened a box of crayons, he smiled and said, "Wow, that smells like childhood." Few things can trigger memories quite like smell. That's because the receptors in the nose send signals to multiple areas of the brain, including the olfactory bulb, which is part of the brain's limbic system. This area is sometimes called the "emotional brain" because this area processes memories and feelings. These receptors take note of seven sensations, generally categorized as camphor, musk, ether, acrid, putrid, mint and flower. The connection between smell and memory is so strong that people can remember a scent with 65% accuracy after a year, while the recall of an image is only about 50% after three months.

While we tend to put more emphasis on the senses of sight, touch and sound when it comes to romantic relationships (How does my partner look? How does my partner feel? How sexy is my partner's voice?), smell is actually one of the most important senses utilized in sexual attraction due to the invisible pheromones that we share. These invisible chemicals are so powerful that they carry a greater influence than we may realize. For evolutionary reasons, both men and women have learned to be attracted to partners with different immune systems than their own, because the combined immune systems help create stronger offspring.

> *"Memories, imagination, old sentiments, and associations are more readily reached through the sense of smell than through any other channel."*
>
> *– Dr. Oliver Wendell Holmes*

Women are more sensitive to the smell of pheromones than men, and they affect a woman's love biochemical receptors. In his book *The Owners Manual of the Brain,* Dr. Pierce J. Howard shows that pheromones can even be at the root of a romantic disconnect, even after a relationship has started. The make-up of many birth control pills causes women to be attracted to men with similar immune systems, as detected via pheromones. But after a long period of time, including into marriage, a woman may go off her birth control, and suddenly wonder why she was ever attracted to such a man.

Given the strong connection between smell and emotion, it's important to be aware of what smells work and don't work for your partner. For instance, Napoleon specifically asked his wife Josephine not to bathe for the two weeks before he returned from battle because he liked her natural scent. Would she have done this if he hadn't asked?

> "We crave love; we go through withdrawal from love; we relapse into love; we pursue love at all costs."
>
> - Dr. Helen Fisher

As a side note, did you realize that the vagina doesn't need to be douched? As Eve Ensler, playwright of The Vagina Monologues says, "My vagina doesn't need to be cleaned up. It smells good already." She's right; the vagina is the cleanest place in the female body with a perfect pH balance that is self-cleaning.

It can be confusing to understand what smells work for some and not for others because our own sense of scents is so engrained in our minds that we may not even realize the psychological aspects at play. What may remind you of great sex could remind your partner of a bad break up so, if in doubt, go for the cleanest smells possible as a starting point and build up from there.

NEURO-CISE: SMELL, DUO

- ♥ While beautiful to look at, make sure the scent of flowers is a positive experience. Don't place them near ripening fruit or vegetables, as they will wilt quicker.

- ♥ Don't use scented candles during a meal because their smell could conflict with the aroma of the food.

- ♥ Experiment with soaps, lotions, shampoos and essential oils to find out which ones you and your partner find most pleasing.

- ♥ Shower with your partner and enjoy the purity of their clean smell.

- ♥ Put potpourri sachets in your undies drawer.

- ♥ Spray flower scents around your bedroom before sleep to promote more positive dreams. Clinical trials have shown that the smell of lavender can help in insomnia, anxiety, stress, and post-operative pain, according to a report from Maryland University.

Only Your Nose Knows

Aromatherapy can be a great way to enhance intimacy. In studies conducted by the Smell and Taste Treatment and Research Foundation in Chicago, the scent of pumpkin pie was found to increase penile blood flood by 40% while increasing sexual desire in women as well. Who says you have to wait until Thanksgiving? Here's a list of additional scents to keep in mind, as they have been known to increase sex drive:

♥ Basil   ♥ Juniper

♥ Cedarwood   ♥ Lavender

♥ Sage   ♥ Patchouli

♥ Ginger   ♥ Sandalwood

♥ Geranium   ♥ Ylang Ylang

♥ Jasmine   ♥ Vanilla

Taste of Heaven

Of course, the pleasures of the nose are matched only by the pleasures of the tongue. Like rock 'n roll, taste is big and bold and exhilarating. Can you imagine a life without knowing the pleasures of chocolate, fresh strawberries or seafood? Well, thanks to friendly little chemical receptors on the tongue, roof of mouth and throat, you don't have to. For the most part, the tip of tongue reads sweetness and the back of the tongue is sensitive to bitterness with salty and sour receptors found on the top and sides of the tongue. The signals move along through the limbic system, which also reads the messages for odors. Given the proximity of the pathways for taste and smell, it's little wonder that there is a symbiotic relationship between the two.

"The sensation of flavor is actually a combination of taste and smell," said Tom Finger, a professor at the University of Colorado-Denver Medical School. "If you hold your nose and start chewing a jelly bean, taste is limited, but open your nose midway through chewing and then you suddenly recognize apple or watermelon." This explains why taste is affected when a head cold renders a person stuffed up and unable to smell. Conversely, a scented candle burning on the dining room table will affect the taste of the meal.

While it's usually true that denying one sense enhances the others, we can see now that this doesn't pertain to the relationship between smell and taste. However, taste will be greatly enhanced by removing other senses, most notably sight. It can be extremely erotic to enhance the sense of taste with blindfold play. Take turns with a blindfold, and feed each other some tasty foods such as juicy fruits or fine cheeses.

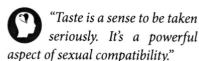

"Taste is a sense to be taken seriously. It's a powerful aspect of sexual compatibility."

– *Dr. Pepper Schwartz*

It's also incredibly erotic to intimately explore your partner's body with your tongue without the aid of vision. Pay attention to taste of their kiss. Savor the sweetness of their sweat. Lovingly perform oral sex, not as a means to intercourse but as an act of sensory exploration.

Speaking of oral sex, the flavor of semen and vaginal juices can be influenced by the foods we eat. If you're going to explore the flavors of the body, the best thing to do is to have a fruit-filled diet leading up to the adult playtime, as the natural sugars enhance the flavors in both sexes. Coffee, beer, garlic, onion, and milk products all create less pleasurable flavors, generally speaking. Smokers tend to taste the most bitter, which is another good reason to give up smoking.

Light My Fire

Stories about aphrodisiacs and their abilities to increase sexual desire have been around for decades and run the gamut from seeds to sweets to serpents.

There's plenty of debate on whether there are any true aphrodisiacs but there are certainly reasons why some may work as triggers for sexual enhancement. The most powerful aphrodisiacs work on both physiological and psychological levels. The smell of jasmine, perhaps, could be a physiological aphrodisiac which also brings you back psychologically to that incredible night when you made love in the garden by jasmine bushes.

Many of the foods heralded as aphrodisiacs may simply be considered sexual because of their shape. Consider the phallic shape of carrots, cucumber, bananas, leaks, zucchini, and licorice, or the female sexual organ design of clams, mangos, figs, kiwi, artichoke, peaches and passion fruit. The act of eating them can feel sexual given the way they look, or the fact that they are juicy, messy or moist on the tongue.

There are a few foods, however, that have caught the attention of scientific researchers with the authentic enhancements they provide. For instance:

♥ A stalk of crunchy celery is packed with two pheromones that can help men attract women, according to Dr. Alan Hirsch, a neurologist and psychiatrist who has devoted over 25 years of research to the science of smell and taste.

♥ Vanilla ice cream can boost your libido and can make your orgasm more powerful. A study conducted at Chicago's Smell and Taste Treatment & Research Foundation found that when men smell the scent of vanilla it reduces their inhibitions.

♥ The American Dietetic Association reports that Brazil nuts can help keep sperm cells healthy. If you prefer almonds, you're in luck as they are also libido-boosting vitamin E.

♥ Blueberries are Mother Nature's original potency food for men with erectile problems. Professor Mary Ellen Camire at the University of Maine reports that they are loaded with soluble fiber, which helps push excess cholesterol through the digestive system and they are packed with compounds that help relax blood vessels, improving circulation all through the body.

♥ The naughty looking banana can help your body produce sex hormones a few hours before getting it on and it converts carbs into energy so it will give you more endurance between the sheets.

♥ The Journal of Sexual Medicine reports that one cube of dark chocolate daily can lead to greater desire and better overall sexual function.

♥ Cherries are sweet and tasty, but also stimulate pheromone production and have potassium that is essential for producing sexual hormones.

♥ Cucumber is a phallic looking food that arouses women with its aroma as well as its taste. Nutritionally, it provides several nutrients essential for sexual health, including Vitamin C and a mineral called manganese.

♥ Strawberries are luscious to look at and delicious to eat, but they are also a high source of vitamin C and are rich in antioxidants that benefit the heart and help lower cholesterol.

♥ Ladies chewing on black licorice found it to enhance love and lust as it contains plant estrogens and stimulates the sex glands, bringing oxygen to the female genitals 40% faster.

Are They Or Aren't They?

Many believe that alcohol is an aphrodisiac, but it doesn't raise sexual interest as much as it lowers inhibitions. Quickly absorbed by the digestive system and the bloodstream, drinking taints judgment, impairs memory, creates mood swings, and reduces control of motor skills. Sexually, these consequences diminish performance, healthy decision-making, and the quality of relationships. It also has the ability to undermine self-esteem, which hinders sexual pleasure. Doubts about love, attractiveness, and worthiness run amuck. And let's not forget that too much booze can mean too little sexual sensation, including impotence. Alcohol is haunted by an aphrodisiacal paradox. When the edge of "just enough" is crossed, the substance goes from sexually good to sexually bad.

A different but similar paradox is found in medicines created to treat erectile dysfunction. Some men consider the introduction of Viagra to be the greatest medical breakthrough in the history of time. As grandiose as that sounds, it gives some insight into the importance virility holds in the minds of many. Proclaimed by some sexologists as "the greatest aphrodisiac of our time," Viagra and its brethren are certainly noteworthy, but the medicine at work doesn't exactly fall within the formal definition of the word.

Sildenafil nitrate is the drug commonly known as Viagra, Levitra and Cialis. People view it as an aphrodisiac, but clinically there is no evidence that this impotence treatment changes sexual desire at all. Without the component of desire, sex is like digestion. The system produces a physical change (penis engorges with blood), but the physiological component that defines a true aphrodisiac is left out. Now where is the pleasure in that?

I Know This Much Is True

All of the senses are wondrous, but the sixth sense is mysterious. Intuition is like a great jazz band. It relies on improvisation, mystery and surprise and it also depends on all the other senses to play along. The study of intuition is still in its infancy but there's no denying the important role it plays in our daily lives.

Even those with no interest in talking about psychic abilities or the more esoteric definitions of the sixth sense can't deny that at one time or another a thought, idea, decision or inspiration seemed to spring forth without cause or effort. An impulse to take action came out of nowhere. Sometimes we listen to these messages and sometimes we don't, but many times we can trace our path back to that instinct when the "ah-ha" moment presented itself.

For instance, perhaps you're single and you walk your dog on the exactly same route every night after dinner. Suddenly one night you feel the urge to go a different way for no explicable reason. Why would you suddenly want to turn on a side street when you've always taken the main road? On this night, you decide to trust your gut which leads you to meeting the love of your life when you cross paths at an intersection neither one of you had ever seen before.

How did you receive this message? It wasn't random or accidental. It was a clear thought that came out of the blue, fully formulated and requesting that you follow its lead and doing so lead to an answer to a question you didn't even realize you were asking!

While many studies have been done, acts of intuition have yet to set off a sensor spotlighting the corner of the brain where this magic takes place. While the other senses have their clearly established and noted channels of communication in the brain, perhaps intuition and the other aspects of the sixth sense are actually located in the mind. The interpretation of various signals incorporating brain signals as well as the subconscious memories, thoughts, desires and emotions all click in place and offer a solution to a problem that only the subconscious has been paying attention to while the conscious mind deals with the tangible world.

> "Intuition will tell the thinking mind where to look next."
>
> – Dr. Jonas Salk

I don't have the answer to where intuition lives in the brain but I <u>do</u> know how it can be enhanced. It doesn't require magic spells, Tarot cards or a crystal ball. The only thing needed to strengthen the sixth sense is a willingness to slow down and listen.

Life is moving very fast these days. Not only are we juggling fast food, a cell phone and a steering wheel while flying along the highway, but we're also processing the various conversations we've had and/or need to have with our co-workers, partner, kids, friends, and family while also keeping a running tally of daily successes and failures as the TICK TOCK TICK TOCK of the life clock taunts us at every turn. More. Faster. Bigger. Better. More. More. MORE.

And now I have the nerve to suggest that you slow down? Who has time to slow down? You do and you need to take it.

I was speaking with spiritual leader and energy guru Gurutej about this portion of the book and she laughed, saying, "Life is not a race. Most people are terrified of dying but they live like they can't get to the end fast enough." This feels absolutely true and the only way to change it is to make the decision to slow down.

Gurutej also said, "Miracles are not something that happen, they are something you become aware of." I think some people are surprised by their intuition and the ways in which it can pay off. When success arrives, sometimes it feels like a miracle happening outside of you, and you happened to be lucky enough to catch it. But what experts in this field suggest is that the miracle was there for you all the time, you just needed to fully embrace the potential of your clear mind and its intuitive power. Take the time to let it breathe. Literally.

NEURO-CISE: BREATH, SOLO

We all take breathing for granted until it becomes compromised. Honestly, how often do you think about the fact that you're breathing? And are you aware of HOW you breathe?

Here's a simple breathing exercise that can help clear the mind. Like a lot of things that are good for the body, it's incredibly simple but possibly something you have never considered.

Alternative nostril breathing is a Yogic exercise where you alternate which nostril you are inhaling and exhaling through in order to focus oxygen on the two sides of the brain: the left nostril is thought to be calming while the right nostril is energizing. Breathing through your left nostril will access the right "feeling" hemisphere of your brain, and breathing in through your right nostril, will access the left "analyzing" hemisphere of your brain. Consciously alternating your breath between either nostril will allow you to activate and access your whole brain. The flip side of course is that *single* nostril breathing can be used to activate just the left "analyzing" or just right "feeling" side of your brain for specific situations.

♥ Ideally you would be sitting comfortably with minimal distractions.

♥ Exhale fully and then close off the right nostril with your finger or thumb.

♥ Inhale through the left nostril and then close off that nostril.

♥ Fully exhale through the right nostril and then inhale through the right nostril before closing it.

♥ Now repeat this action, moving back and forth, inhaling and exhaling out of both sides.

♥ Continue as long as it's comfortable, with nine full repetitions.

There are many health benefits to incorporating this kind of simple breathing exercise into your life. It improves brain function and revitalizes you while also calming an agitated mind by soothing the nervous system. This calmer mental state allows for more clarity, which in turns works as an invitation to intuition and creativity.

NEURO-CISE: BREATH, DUO

Synchronized breathing while touching each other is easy to implement into your daily life and will give you the added benefits of optimal levels of oxytocin.

♥ You can breathe together while standing and hugging.

♥ Laying down and cuddling.

♥ With one person's head in the other's lap.

♥ Sitting or lying back to back.

As long as your bodies are touching, you can breathe in synchronicity inhaling and exhaling together and sharing your life force energy.

By taking the time to match your breathing, you are creating a deeper connection while relaxing that will result in bringing you both into the present.

All Together Now

Our senses are the instruments that bring the outside music in. What we see, hear, taste, smell, and feel paints our picture of the world. At the same time, these senses can be used to embed us deeply into the sensory circuits of our partner's brain. We are so lucky to have this astonishing toolbox built into our brains that can help us solve relationship problems, attract new mates and create peace of mind. Cultivating our senses is enjoyable, useful and free!

You can take stock of what you're presenting and make sure it is the message you want to send. Do you have all the tools you need to smooth out any rough edges and make yourself even more inviting? Do you have the power to deepen the sensory

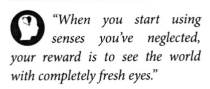

"When you start using senses you've neglected, your reward is to see the world with completely fresh eyes."

– Barbara Sher

connection with the ones you love? The next step in your intimate evolution is to enhance The Mind, Body and Energy Experience.

CHAPTER FIVE
The Mind, Body and Energy Experience

To be fully engaged in life, we must become aware of the extraordinary connection between our mental state and our physical being. Everything we do relies on neurons communicating with one another, electrical impulses and chemical signals carrying messages across different parts of the brain as well as between the brain and the rest of the nervous system. The body and mind work together to heighten all our experiences, our love and sex lives included.

Scientists have also discovered that emotions have a physical place in the brain. Anger, happiness, sadness, fear - each has a specific neural circuitry that has evolved over millions of years. Interestingly, many dichotomous emotions reside in the same place. For example, fear and anger come from the same area of the brain, which is the root of the "fight or flight" response. Similarly, pain and pleasure are also roommates. Studies have shown that people who enjoy BDSM (Bondage, Domination/Discipline, Sadism and Masochism) ignite the same areas of their brains for both the pleasure and the pain they experience.

Emotional Hurt, Physical Pain

When people feel emotional pain, it triggers the same areas of the brain as physical pain. Why is this? Going back to our initial definition of feelings, the body responds to the messages of the mind. This applies to a broken heart as much as a broken toe.

Our body responds to our thoughts and feelings. Below is a just a short list of some of the physical conditions that can indicate our emotional health is out of balance:

- ♥ Back pain
- ♥ Chest pain
- ♥ Constipation
- ♥ Exhaustion
- ♥ Headaches
- ♥ High blood pressure

- ♥ Insomnia
- ♥ Palpitations
- ♥ Sexual problems
- ♥ Stiff neck
- ♥ Upset stomach
- ♥ Weight changes

Alan Fogel, Ph.D., explored this phenomenon for *Psychology Today* ("Where Does Emotion Hurt In The Body?" 2012) with a series of insightful questions, most notably this one about tripping over a box someone left behind, "If my brain sends me the signal that I broke my toe and I can feel it *in* my toe, where does my brain place the emotional pain of anger I have for the guy that left the box in the hallway?" More directly, "Where does emotional pain hurt?"

Fogel wonders if emotional pain might reside in the area of the body that represents that unexpressed emotion. For instance, in the example of a toe stubbed on a box left in the hallway, the decision to not yell at the culprit may result in tension in the neck, throat and jaw because the desired expression was not taken, so the muscle that would have otherwise been exercised becomes tense. So, really, saying someone is a "pain in the neck" is more truth than cliché.

Using this logic, is "heartbreak" a real thing? Some researchers believe so. The feeling of love is partly created by vagal-parasympathetic activation, which promotes an easy and relaxed integration of breathing and heart rate. When this comfortable feeling is challenged by deception or a break up, the sympathetic nervous system responds the same as if it were a physical threat. Since the safety was felt in the chest area, the body may go into protection mode, thereby causing shoulders to hunch into a downcast posture as if to protect the chest and the heart from further pain.

It is important to become aware of where emotional pain resides in our bodies because the location may hold the key to releasing the pain. To improve your emotional and physical health, keep these basic goals in mind:

- ♥ Don't repress, deny or ignore your feelings.

- ♥ Express your feelings in appropriate ways.

- ♥ Maintain a positive outlook.

- ♥ Develop resilience.

- ♥ Practice relaxation techniques.

- ♥ Take care of your body with healthy nutrition and exercise.

Take a moment to pay attention to your body. Do you have a physical pain that isn't related to a known injury or ailment? If so, how might it be related to unresolved emotional pain? There is a valuable technique that I've used for myself and with my clients called Body, Mind Dialog which can help to release the pain.

NEURO-CISE: MIND, BODY DIALOG, SOLO

- ♥ Get into a comfortable position sitting at your computer or have a pad and pen at the ready, without any other distractions. Close your eyes and take a few deep breaths to relax.

♥ Become aware of the part of your body where you experience pain or discomfort and give it an identity, such as a teenager behaving badly that shows up unexpectedly and is disruptive.

♥ Give the identity a voice as you open up your eyes and start writing. Ask questions about why it is hurting you, such as: Why are you here? What do you want? How can I make you go away?

♥ Be open to the answers you may receive from your body and write them down without trying to edit or analyze them.

♥ Keep writing until you feel that you have learned something new about your body and pain, hopefully with a positive conclusion.

One of my clients wrote a dialog with her vagina because she was experiencing pain during intercourse. When she read her script to me at my office, I could tell how upset she was by what she had learned from this exercise. She was crying as she read the words, "I don't like the way your boyfriend treats you and I'm not going to let him in." She asked me what she should do next and I told her to thank her vagina entity for telling her the truth. This exercise revealed what her body knew and her mind was afraid to admit.

> *"The best way to get rid of the pain is to feel the pain. And when you feel the pain and go beyond it, you'll see there's a very intense love that is wanting to awaken itself."*
>
> *– Dr. Deepak Chopra*

Exploring a Holistic Approach

By definition, the word "holistic" relates to the whole mind and body system. The Chopra Center defines holistic in its original sense, as related to *Wholeness*. Dr. Deepak Chopra's guide to holistic health emphasizes the energy and information you take in through your mind and the influence of the sensory organs on your body and spirit. The secret is to live in wholeness now, cultivating a lifestyle that nurtures all aspects of your life – including your physical and emotional health, relationships, success in fulfilling your dreams and desires, personal growth, and spiritual connection.

Dr. Daniel J. Siegel is a clinical professor of psychiatry, director of the Mindsight Institute and author of several books on the brain including, *The Mindful Brain* and *Brainstorm*, whose work examines the energy flow that happens in the body and how the sharing of this energy and information creates and defines relationships. As he states, "How your heart is beating, what hormones are racing through your bloodstream, how your immune system is functioning ... all these bodily functions influence feelings and thoughts and memories."

In one study of patients with a common cold, he found that doctors that added a single comment that expressed empathy – "This must be really hard for you ... you have a school exam that you can't do" – got over their cold one day sooner than those patients who didn't receive the empathetic comment. What this underscores is the growing belief that treating only the symptoms is not nearly enough.

Applying this holistic approach to relationship building comes down to one word: awareness. When conflict comes up, it's important to step back from the immediate problem to see how the larger scope of things is effecting the moment. Are you fighting with your partner because you have unresolved conflict with your boss? Is the argument over money really an expression of self-punishment for losing a bet on last week's football game? Are you denying your partner sex tonight because dirty dishes were left in the sink this morning?

In the heat of the moment it can be difficult to allow enough breathing room to see things clearly, so it's important to recognize your own triggers and to be very careful with your words, as words can be a lethal

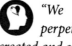 *"We are always in a perpetual state of being created and creating ourselves."*

– Dr. Dan Siegel

weapon. Nothing can ever be unsaid, so be sure to speak from a place of clarity.

Dr. Brenda Wade, author of *Love Lessons: A Guide to Transforming Relationships* uses the analogy of a car to explain the interaction between emotion and energy. "When you take the time to experience and express your emotions, energy is released. On the other hand, unexpressed emotion becomes blocked, stuck energy. This is kind of like a car that needs a tune-up to be fuel-efficient and to run smoothly."

NEURO-CISE: EMOTIONAL TUNE UP, SOLO

Dr. Wade recommends we use this five-minute emotional tune-up every day.

1. Take a deep breath.

2. Place your hand on your heart.

3. Ask, "What am I feeling today?"

4. Let yourself say the emotions out loud or write them down. The key is to experience and express your feelings.

5. What do you need to do, be or have to feel emotionally supported and connected to yourself and those in your life?

Hello, Chakras

Perhaps just reading that heading caused you to roll your eyes. A discussion of energy centers may seem as credible to you as a unicorn sighting, but I ask you to bear with me. If the scientific foundation of the previous discussion of emotions manifesting physically in the body intrigued you at all, you're already half way to understanding chakras.

 Emotional energy is our fuel."

- Dr. Brenda Wade

The word "chakra" means "wheel" in the Sanskrit (ancient Hindu) language and according to beliefs that go back over 5000 years, there are seven energy wheels that run down the center of our body, which energy flows through. These are the chakras, and they are all interconnected to light, sound and color. Understanding the chakras allows us to understand the relationship between our consciousness and our physical body because blocked energy in our chakras can often lead to illness, while unencumbered chakras lead to wellbeing.

The Taoist view of emotions is that they are forms of energy rooted in the organ system as described by Chinese medicine. When the flow of energy through our organ systems is unbalanced, our emotions may manifest into negative ones such as fear, anger or sadness. Healing is possible through freeing energy with the mind-body connection.

If you've ever felt a sudden lump in your throat, butterflies in your stomach or an aching heart, then you have experienced your chakras trying to communicate with you. They are giving you signals that you need to pay attention to; otherwise they will become unbalanced and can possibly cause emotional or physical discomfort, pain or even disease. Let's explore each of the Chakras in greater detail.

1st Root Chakra (Red)

This chakra is located in the base of the spine and coccygeal area that supports the anus.

Much like a root anchors a tree in the physical world, our emotional core keeps our mental world grounded. When our Root Chakra is open it gives us a sense of security, of being in control of our life and our destiny.

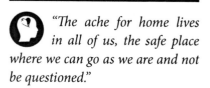

"The ache for home lives in all of us, the safe place where we can go as we are and not be questioned."

– Dr. Maya Angelou

When our Root Chakra is blocked, we may feel insecure, guilty or ashamed and have a sense of not belonging.

NEURO-CISE: ROOT CHAKRA, DUO

- ♥ Sit opposite your partner with legs crossed at the ankles, hold hands and look at each other as you tell your partner what makes you feel safe, grounded and confident.

- ♥ Hip circles will open up your Solar plexus, Sacral and Root Chakras. Stand up and face each other, or do it alone. With your knees bent slightly, push your pelvis forward, still keeping the knees bent. Now rotate your pelvis in large circles clock-wise, 10 times and then anti-clock wise 10 times. Keep your head and feet still while only moving your pelvis area. Focus on opening up your sensuality.

- ♥ Put your hand on your Root Chakra. Face your partner and finish this sentence "I feel secure when you ..."

NEURO-CISE: ROOT CHAKRA, SOLO

- ♥ Stomping can be fun to do outside as you stomp your feet on the ground until you feel more grounded.

- ♥ Root squeezing can be done while sitting, lying down or standing with your knees slightly apart. Then tighten and pull up your sphincter muscles as tightly as you can. Hold tightened for at least five seconds, then relax for at least ten seconds and repeat five times to strengthen the anal sphincter muscles.

2nd Sacral Chakra (Orange)

Located in the ovaries and testes that produce various sex hormones, this chakra is connected to our reproductive capacity and sexual desire.

When our Sacral Chakra is open, we feel creative, free of guilt or shame, and emotionally and sexually fulfilled with a sense of abundance. When the Sacral Chakra is blocked, it can result in feelings of frustration especially in relationships, lack of sexual energy or desire, and blocked creativity.

NEURO-CISE: SACRAL CHAKRA, DUO

♥ Sit opposite your partner with legs crossed at the ankles, lean in, hold hands and look at each other. Take turns speaking and listening as you share the following. When do you feel creative, sexually open and uninhibited?

♥ Put your hand on your Sacral Chakra and tell your partner what he/she does to turn you on the most.

NEURO-CISE: SACRAL CHAKRA, SOLO

♥ Belly dancing is one of the best physical activities to open up the Sacral Chakra, but if belly dancing is not your style, try some pelvic thrusting movements to get the blood flowing to your pelvic regions.

♥ The Cobra Pose is an ancient yoga pose that is excellent for the mind, body and energy experience, but especially opening up the sacral chakra. Lie face down on the floor with palms flat and fingers spread beneath your shoulders. Then push your upper body off the floor as you tilt your head toward the ceiling and arching your back while your lower body remains against the floor Once your arms are fully extended, close your eyes, hold the position for three full breaths, then release and open up your eyes. Repeat five times. A little time spent in cobra pose can go a long way towards alleviating anxiety and stress.

3rd Solar Plexus Chakra (Yellow)

Located in the upper abdomen in the stomach area, this chakra is related to the digestive system and is also known as our "Seat of Emotions." It is our energy center for power, which includes anger and laughter.

When our Solar Plexus Chakra is open, we feel powerful, confident and self-assured, like we have control of our lives. When it is blocked, we feel insecure and introverted, which often leads to anxiety and depression.

NEURO-CISE: SOLAR PLEXUS CHAKRA, DUO

♥ Practice forgiveness. The word "forgive" literally means "to give up," "to give away." Forgiveness is a form of unburdening, removing emotional clutter that can keep you blocked from experiencing giving and receiving love. You can start a weekly forgiveness ritual by forgiving yourself for things you did that you wish you hadn't done. If you are in a relationship, you can write a forgiveness letter by letting your partner know what he or she did to hurt you. You can even forgive someone silently by saying, "I forgive you for what you have done to me knowingly or unknowingly to hurt me."

♥ Share your personal power with your partner by letting him or her know your strengths and your weaknesses. Then work together to help each other develop the weaknesses into strengths.

NEURO-CISE: SOLAR PLEXUS CHAKRA, SOLO

♥ Use a hula-hoop to open up your Solar Plexus Chakra by pushing your stomach forward as the hoop moves across it. Then push the hoop back when it moves across your back. Keep moving your waist in circular motions to release your solar plexus energy until the hoop falls. Then try spinning it in the opposite direction.

♥ Dancing the twist to your favorite oldies music from the 1960's can open up the Solar Plexus Chakra without needing any props. Just put one foot in front of the other so that you can shift your body weight from the front to the back leg. Bend your elbows at your side slightly and start to twist from your waist from left to right leaning slightly forward with weight on your front leg, then lean slightly backwards, as you continue to twist with weight on your back leg.

4th Heart Chakra (Green)

Located in the center of the chest and just above the heart, this energy center is related to the immune system as well as being part of the endocrine system. Key issues involving the Heart Chakra involve compassion, love and spirituality.

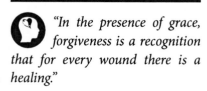 *"In the presence of grace, forgiveness is a recognition that for every wound there is a healing."*

– Dr. Deepak Chopra

When your Heart Chakra is open, you love yourself and others without judgment. You are compassionate and feel balanced. When your Heart Chakra is blocked, you feel unable to give and receive love; you lack peace of mind and find it hard to trust anyone.

NEURO-CISE: HEART CHAKRA, DUO

♥ Become your Heart Chakra and express to your partner how you want to be loved. Ask your partner to tell you how he/she wants you to love them back.

♥ Place your prominent hand on each other's heart, close your eyes and tune into your partner's heartbeat. Breath in and out in a slow steady rhythm together and feel the connection between your life force energies expand your heart to let more love in to your life.

NEURO-CISE: HEART CHAKRA, SOLO

♥ Practice hugging people who you care about, regularly.

♥ Do the breaststroke in a pool or even as part of your exercise regimen out of water to open up your Heart Chakra.

♥ Give yourself at least three positive affirmations every day. They can be for love, health, success, abundance or any other goal you may have. Always start with "I am ..." and then fill in the blank as if it has already happened. For example, "I am loved", "I am in great health", or "I am a confident and positive person worthy of the success I have."

5th Throat Chakra (Sky Blue)

The Throat Chakra is located in the neck, throat and thyroid gland responsible for our body's metabolism. This energy center influences our communication and how we express ourselves so that we are heard the way we want to be perceived.

When your Throat Chakra is open, you have the ability to express yourself honestly and creatively so that people hear and understand what you have to say. You are also good at listening and are able to give constructive advice. When your Throat Chakra is blocked, you feel insecure about communicating your thoughts for fear of rejection, or fear that people may misunderstand what you say and have a negative perception of you.

NEURO-CISE: THROAT CHAKRA, DUO

- ♥ Put your hand on your Throat Chakra and tell your partner how you feel about your relationship: what is perfect and what would you like to improve.

- ♥ Tell your partner a story about a couple that lived happily ever after and make sure that the characters have your names.

NEURO-CISE: THROAT CHAKRA, SOLO

- ♥ Singing or chanting can open up your Throat Chakra and release the energy you need to better express yourself.

- ♥ Panting like a puppy may sound silly, but it can actually be good for your respiratory system and your Throat Chakra. You don't have to let your tongue fall out of your mouth, but you do have to move your stomach while your throat and chest are relaxed. You can change your exhale to do slow panting or fast panting for a couple of minutes a day, even when you are driving or waiting for the traffic lights to change.

6th Third Eye Chakra (Indigo)

Located in the center of the forehead in between the eyes and linked to the pineal gland that regulates our sleep and waking up, this energy center is connected to our intuition, imagination and ability to think and make decisions.

When our Third Eye Chakra is open we feel intuitive and have the ability to visualize what we want, then execute and reach our goals successfully. When our Third Eye Chakra is blocked, it's hard to imagine anything going right or to follow through on projects, and life can be confusing with lots of conflicts.

NEURO-CISE: THIRD EYE CHAKRA, DUO

- ♥ Face your partner, put your hand on your Third Eye Chakra and finish this sentence: "You don't know I ..." Then it's your partner's turn to do the same. Be sure to thank each other for sharing.

- ♥ Share a time when you listened to your intuition and it worked, and name a time you didn't follow your intuition and you wish that you had.

NEURO-CISE: THIRD EYE CHAKRA, SOLO

- ♥ Guided imagery through all of your senses can result in deep emotions. Make your imagery as vivid as possible because our bodies do not discriminate between sensory images in our mind and reality. If you imagine that you are happy and satisfied, your brain will automatically believe it and your body will respond.

- ♥ You can also create a vision board if it helps you with this exercise. Simply collect a collage of pictures and post them on a board to help you envision your future outcome. For example, if you are looking for love, find a picture of your perfect mate and add it to your board. If you want a dream house or job, find a picture that represents what you are looking for and place it on your board, which should be on display in a prominent place where you can see it every day.

♥ Child's pose is a wonderful way to stretch your body and open up your Third Eye Chakra every day. Get into a kneeling position on the floor with your buttocks resting on your heels. Then lean your upper body forward with your arms stretched out in front of you so that your stomach is resting on top of your thighs and your head is on the floor. Even if you only do this pose a few times a day, the benefits will be noticeable for your neck, shoulders, back and hips as it releases strain and tension from these areas. It also flexes the body's internal organs, stretches the spine and calms the mind.

> "The intuitive mind is a sacred gift and the rational mind is a faithful servant. We have created a society that honors the servant and has forgotten the gift."
>
> - Albert Einstein

7th Crown Chakra (Deep Violet)

Located at the crown of the head, the Crown Chakra is considered to be the chakra of pure consciousness and wisdom. It is attached to the central nervous system via the hypothalamus.

When your Crown Chakra is open, you feel like you have found your mission in life, taken the right path and that your journey will make a significant impact on the world. When your Crown Chakra is blocked, you question your knowledge and fear the unknown. You are skeptical. Your life's mission is unclear and your personal growth is stunted.

NEURO-CISE: CROWN CHAKRA, DUO

♥ Put your hand on your Crown Chakra and tell your partner where you would like to see your relationship in the future (1-5 years) time.

♥ Share what you can do together to feel spiritually alive and connected.

NEURO-CISE: CROWN CHAKRA, SOLO

♥ This stretching exercise will open up your Crown, Third Eye and Throat Chakras. Lie down flat on your back on a hard surface like the floor with your feet touching. Then raise your head, shoulders and back to a seated position. Place your hands on your hips or on the floor if you need support and tip your head back looking up to the sky. Breathe deeply through your nose and exhale through your mouth five times. Focus on opening up your mind.

♥ Create a movie in your mind where you are the star, writer, director and producer, constantly editing and rewriting your script and deciding how you want it to end. Choose which characters play lead, supporting or extra roles in your movie. Creative visualization is a performance-enhancement technique that can be a confidence booster, natural anti-depressant, stress reliever, motivator and inspiration that will open up your highest chakra, and reach your goals.

And Now ... Tantra

Tantra is an enormous topic with many facets, but I've learned over the years that there are a few elements that are easy to understand and are immediately helpful.

Margot Anand, best-selling author of *The Art of Everyday Ecstasy*, describes the power of Tantra this way, "Truly, at the peak of orgasm, we pierce through the illusion of fragmentation and separation, and glimpse the unity and interconnectedness of all beings. And through the other–our partner–we fall in love with life."

Tantric sex has a rejuvenating effect. It affects brain chemistry by igniting the endocrine glands for more HGH, serotonin, DHEA, testosterone and oxytocin. (For a more thorough overview of the various brain chemicals at work, please see *Chapter Three, BrainGasm: Understanding the Science of Love & Sex*). Tantra can also improves sexual health, and many scientific studies point to physical benefits such as stimulated blood circulation, body detoxification, and strengthened cardiovascular, endocrine, immune and nervous functions.

What Tantra Is

Many people are unclear about what Tantra is and what it is not. Tantra is not a religion, a sexual cult, a new age spiritual philosophy, exhibitionism, swinging or sex therapy. And there are different kinds of Tantra including White Tantra, which directs energy to expand our spiritual awareness (His Holiness the Dalai Lama practices White Tantra), but you can also practice White Tantra while meditating or doing yoga with your partner. Black Tantra is the opposite as it directs energy to manipulate another person sexually. But we are going to focus on Red Tantra, which directs energy between two lovers that include our thoughts, feelings, physical and sexual actions. Tantra is a Sanskrit word that means "to weave energy", defined by the Yin (feminine) and Yang (masculine) energy between two partners. The sexual energy is often referred to as Kundalini energy that is very powerful and can be used:

- ♥ For a couple to heal a hurt relationship.

- ♥ For women, Tantra can empower and fulfill their sensual needs.

- ♥ For men, it can open up a whole new world to intimacy and it can give them the tools to become multi-orgasmic.

- ♥ For couples, it's also an opportunity to create a more meaningful and intimate connection.

- ♥ Mindful loving.

- ♥ An art.

- ♥ Sexual enlightenment.

A Brief History

About 5,000 years ago, Lord Shiva's followers developed 112 methods of meditation, through which one could enter the state of super-consciousness. Some of them included the act of sex. Lord Shiva's symbol, the Lingam ("the wand of light") represents the penis and rests in a Yoni ("the sacred place") that represents the vagina. Very simply explained, the entire path of Tantra is the harmonious union of the masculine and feminine principles in all of us.

 "We will make love an art and we will love like artists."

– Marianne Williamson

Yin and Yang

Like most forces throughout the world, light and dark, hot and cold, wet and dry, positive and negative, there are two essential principles to lovemaking: yin and yang. Yin means feminine and Yang means masculine.

We all have yin and yang attributes and qualities. It would be easy to say that all men are sexual, strong and assertive and all women are sensual, sensitive and submissive, but we know that's not true.

Lots of women are sexual, strong and assertive and many men are sensual, sensitive and enjoy being submissive. A healthy person has a combination of yin and yang attributes and qualities, and looks for someone to complement them, not complete them.

To experience the full enjoyment of Tantric lovemaking, the male and female forces must be balanced in harmony. For example, deep kissing and tender kissing is a perfect combination of yin and yang. Let's face it, if you only kissed your partner tenderly, it would become boring, predictable and lack sexuality. On the other hand, if you only kissed your partner deeply, you would probably have sore lips and get bored with that, too.

We don't always need a big production when it comes to lovemaking, but we do need to be prepared for Tantric sex. When you and your partner have the right ambience, you will have a greater opportunity to enjoy a fulfilling and

"The beauty and wisdom of Tantra is that it enhances sexuality as a doorway to the 'ecstatic mind of great bliss.'"

- Margot Anand

romantic sexual experience. One of the best ways to set the mood for love is to incorporate all five of your senses in your lovemaking. If you don't utilize even one of your senses, you deprive yourself of 20% of the pleasure! That's why it's best to prepare something to enhance all five of your senses prior to your lovemaking session.

The six basic elements of Tantra are: breath, movement, sound, muscle lock, intention and attention.

Breath

Breath is the essence of life, and there is no better way to energize the body than to increase your intake of oxygen. Breathing in through the mouth produces an energy charge and breathing out of the mouth releases emotions. That's why when a person cries, they have to breathe through their mouth. Nostril breathing holds in the energy charge and it enhances sexual control.

NEURO-CISE: BREATHING, SOLO

Make a commitment to take long deep breaths while you are doing every day activities, such as driving, watching TV, reading, taking a bath and so on. When you make love, slow down your normal breathing pattern because, the faster the breath flows, the faster the orgasm.

Stress Breath
When you are stressed out, inhale 4 breaths then exhale 4 breaths.

Cannon Breath

When you are upset, inhale one long deep breath and then exhale it with force as if it were shooting out of a cannon.

Dragon Breath

When you are angry, inhale 4 breaths and then stick your tongue out as you exhale with force. It will make you laugh and you'll forget what you were angry about.

Movement

The energy of touch promotes blood flow, boosts the immune system, and nurtures and arouses via five kinds of touch: healing, romantic, sensual, sexual, or Tantric.

Lack of movement can leave your body feeling tight and tired, restricting energy flow and blocking emotions, especially sexual ones. Even when you visualize parts of your body moving, you are creating physiological sensations.

NEURO-CISE: MOVING, SOLO

- ♥ After you wake up, do some simple stretching exercises to feel more energetic. Add some squats, lunges, push-ups and sit ups to get your body ready for whatever the universe has to throw at you.

- ♥ Park a little further from your destination so that you get a good walk and some fresh air into your lungs.

- ♥ Ride a bike to work or go for a ride on the weekends.

- ♥ Trade the elevator for the stairs.

NEURO-CISE: MOVING, DUO

- ♥ Dance whenever possible with your partner, even if it's just a short sway to the radio in the middle of making dinner.

♥ Hold each other's hands while you do ten lunges together.

♥ Do 5 push-ups on top of your partner and be sure to give them a kiss on the way down.

♥ Go hiking or biking together on the weekends.

Sound
Sound releases energy, including sexual energy during lovemaking. Sound will also amplify sensation, as the sound waves vibrate throughout the body. If you hold back the sounds you feel inside, it will manifest into inhibitions, resentments and anger. Music, laughter and words have the power to heal and arouse, so for your own good health, give yourself permission to express yourself through words, sounds, sighs, cries, shouts and laughter. Hum to yourself every day. Say words you find embarrassing to speak out loud. Make love without restraining your sounds.

NEURO-CISE: CHANTING, SOLO

Chanting is a great way to utilize sound to open chakras: "OHM" for the Crown Chakra, "AH" for the Heart Chakra, and "HOM" for the Sacral Chakra to open. Combining the three will unite these physical areas.

If singing in the shower is more your style, that works too.

NEURO-CISE: SOUNDS OF LOVE, DUO

Making sounds during lovemaking helps to move sexual energy, so your assignment if you choose to accept it is to make passionate love as loudly as possible using sounds to express how you are feeling.

Of course you can be verbal as well as vocal by telling your lover how to please you.

If you are too self-conscious about how you sound, then do your best to praise your partner in and out of the bedroom.

Muscle Lock
The basis for the Tantric muscle lock practice is the Kegel exercise. Kegels can restore muscle tone; increase duration of sexual pleasure and orgasmic awareness.

Achieving simultaneous orgasms with your partner is like doing the Tango. It is a sensual dance made for two people working together, communicating with their bodies and responding to each other's movements.

The PC muscle is the support muscle for the genitals in both men and women. There is a definite correlation between good tone in the PC muscle and orgasmic intensity and control. A quick way to identify the PC muscle is to urinate then stop the flow of urine. After a few repetitions, most people are able to tighten this muscle without involvement of urination.

NEURO-CISE: MUSCLE CONTROL FOR MEN, SOLO

Identify your PC muscle; stop the flow of urine by squeezing the PC muscle, then continue to urinate again. Repeat. This repetition helps increase blood flow to the genitals, increases awareness of feelings in the genitals, restores genital muscle tone and control over orgasms, and heightens the orgasmic experience.

Lingam Lifts
Place a light scarf, handkerchief or tissue on the base of your erect Lingam/penis: then raise it up and down like a weight, using your PC muscle to lift it. Do 20 reps twice a day.

NEURO-CISE: MUSCLE CONTROL FOR WOMEN, SOLO

To locate the PC Muscle, women can insert their finger inside the Yoni (vagina) to feel the inside walls. Look at your genitals in a mirror and watch them contract. Start with 10 of each of the following exercises two times every day.

Slow Kegels

Tighten the PC muscle and hold for a slow count of six seconds. Then relax.

Quick Kegels

Tighten and relax the PC muscle by doing a series of rapid pulsations.

Pulling Push-Outs

Lie down on the floor and take a deep breath. Pull up the entire pelvic floor as though trying to suck water into the Yoni/vagina. Then push out or bear down as if trying to push the water out.

When it is possible to do two sets comfortably, increase the number of repetitions to three. If the muscle seems to tire easily at first, this is normal. Rest between sets for a few minutes and start again. Remember to keep breathing naturally during PC exercises. Doing them during sexual intercourse can be a highly erotic sensation for both of you.

Intention

Where intention goes, energy flows and can take your relationship to a higher level of intimacy. Intention is a vital part of Tantra. It is our intention that helps us to reach our goals. With shared intention comes a deeper heart connection and a higher level of sexual ecstasy.

NEURO-CISE: INTENTION, DUO

- ♥ Give your partner a wish list of 2 things that will heighten a romantic or sexual experience for you both.

- ♥ Put your hand on your partner's Heart Chakra and tell him/ her how you propose to have a deeper heart connection.

- ♥ Share 2 strengths in your relationship. Then tell your partner 1 weakness.

♥ Say, "I intend to show you how I like to be pleasured," and do so.

♥ Ask your partner to show you how he or she likes to be pleasured.

Attention

Attention is all about being 100% present for your partner, focusing on his or her pleasure and sharing your emotions with each other. In the following interactive exercise you will learn how to look into your partner's soul, and how to make love with your full focus. Attention is an essential element to experiencing Tantric bliss and a strong energy connection.

NEURO-CISE: ATTENTION, DUO

Ask your partner if you can look into his or her soul by looking into their eyes. If they say "yes" then look deep into their eyes and tell them what you see. If they say, "no" then invite them to look into your soul by looking into your eyes and ask what they see.

More Than A Simple Touch

Touch is at the center of every sexual experience. It awakens oxytocin, which in turn invites trust and comfort, setting the perfect mood for love, romance and sex.

Neuroscience has given us the tools to understand how and where to touch someone to maximize stimulation. The receptors report physical sensations to the brain, which creates a sensory map. Certain areas of the brain have more touch receptors than others, with the lips, hands, feet, and genitals taking up the largest brain space dedicated to the sensation. Using this information, one can see why holding hands, kissing lips, and stroking a face with fingertips can be very stimulating. The brain has wired these areas to be highly sensitive. In addition to the size of a sensory area, its placement and next-door neighbors can also give us important clues. For example, in the homunculus, the genital area is next door to the foot-sensation area, so a foot massage truly is a form of foreplay.

There are few things more sensual than an erotic massage. This practice has existed for hundreds of years with the intent of releasing tension, heightening levels of communication and creating more intense levels of communication. Varieties of cultures have kept the tradition of erotic, sensual and Tantric massage alive since as far back as 1800 B.C. Aside from literature, hieroglyphics from an ancient Egyptian tomb from 2300 B.C. show what appears to be a foot massage, just like those received by Cleopatra.

We know that there is a symbiotic relationship between our physical lives and our mental wellbeing, so massage is actually one of the most enjoyable ways to improve brain function. Touch and applied pressure to the muscles stimulates the neurotransmitters responsible for sending positive messages to the endocrine, nervous and immune systems. It also reduces levels of the stress hormone cortisol while boosting the feel-good hormones serotonin and dopamine. These changes slow your heart rate, reduce blood pressure, and block pain receptors. Massage has also been known to ease depression, PMS, migraines, labor pains and fibromyalgia.

Massage can also evoke the release of bottled emotions. Being still and vulnerable on the table is just what some people need to uncork their feelings. Many people begin to cry from the sheer emotion of a sexually charged massage session.

The distinction between a Tantric massage and one from a general practitioner is intention and attention. The intention of a Tantric massage is to connect mentally, physically, emotionally, sexually and spiritually. The attention and intent of your movements determine its nature. Ours is a culture starved for touch, and

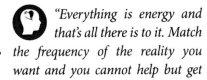

"Everything is energy and that's all there is to it. Match the frequency of the reality you want and you cannot help but get that reality. It can be no other way."

– Albert Einstein

massage is an effective, easy means to feed this hunger.

"Easy?" You may be asking yourself. Perhaps not. Working those muscles and extensively exchanging energy can be exhausting, yet it is easy in the sense that you don't need to be a certified massage therapist to give your partner a memorable Tantric message. The most important component is to focus your energy on pleasing your partner.

NEURO-CISE: TANTRIC MASSAGE, DUO

While it's always nice to have an unplanned foot massage while watching TV or a shoulder rub while doing the dishes, there's nothing quite like the experience of a fully prepared massage, especially one administered by a partner. Let me outline for you how to treat your partner to the ultimate gift.

Have on hand:

- ♥ Oil or lotion
- ♥ Table or bed
- ♥ Stack of blankets
- ♥ Sheets
- ♥ Towels

- ♥ Candles
- ♥ Incense
- ♥ Flowers
- ♥ Smooth finger nails
- ♥ Clean hands
- ♥ Warm wash cloth
- ♥ Bowl of hot water
- ♥ CD Player remote
- ♥ Vibrating mitt or toy

A helpful saying for being present with the person you are massaging is "Be where your hands are." In spiritual programs this is a slogan to keep one's mind on the present task and away from the past or future. In the context of massage, it is not only applicable metaphorically, but literally as well. Focus your positive energy on your partner's body and be in the moment with them. Look at where your hands are. Listen for cues for areas that may need more attention, what feels good, where sensitivity may be located.

Begin by blowing your cool breath with pursed lips over your partner's body, followed by your warm breath with open lips. Then give your partner a light feathery touch using your hair or fingertips from head to toe.

The male chest can handle a firmer stroke and even some kneading, but be very gentle around female breasts, opting for feather strokes. Placing one hand over your partner's heart will create an energetic connection between their heart and wherever your other hand is positioned.

Both men and women have sensation in their nipples (some more than others) so here's your opportunity to find out how sensitive your partner's nipples are by giving them a nipple massage.

NEURO-CISE: HAPPY TECHNIQUES FOR HIM, DUO

Generally speaking, men will have a greater response to gentle but firm and confident touch so approach these exercises with gusto!

Healing Stroke

When it comes to Tantric massage for men, the Healing Stroke is like home base for typing. When you don't know what to type next, your fingers return to ASDFJKL. The Healing Stroke means running the entire palm side of your hand down the underbelly of his shaft and over his scrotum back up and down again. It is an easy maneuver to perform, and frees your second hand to massage his chest, pinch his nipples, or scratch his pubic hair.

Making the Fire

Place the shaft of his lingam between the palms of your hands. Move one hand forward and the other backward. His lingam is like the stick you twist in your hands on a piece of flint to ignite a fire. Start out slowly and gently, but then speed up your rhythm, as he gets more aroused. Make sure to use plenty of oil or lubricant for this technique. Wetter is better!

Spiraling the Stalk

Both hands go in opposite directions in a corkscrew motion over the lingam. One hand twists up while the other hand twists downwards. Increase your rhythm, as he gets more aroused and use lots of oil or lube.

Wet and Wild (Also known as 10 Yoni's)

Now concentrate on just massaging his lingam from the top to the bottom, covering the glans (head) and sliding your hands down to the base with one hand after another in a fluid motion. Do this for at least ten strokes, as many men say that it feels like a woman's yoni/vagina. Don't forget wetter is better!

His Landing Strip/Perineum
(Also known as His Million Dollar Point)

Slowly slide your fingers up and down the perineum from his anus to his scrotum. Feel for a small indentation the size of a pea midway and gently press inward with your thumbs. This area is called the Million Dollar Point in Taoism and many men are able to feel their prostate gland through this point which allows them to experience a much more intense orgasm.

NEURO-CISE: HAPPY TECHNIQUES FOR HER, DUO

While you may be tempted to use massage oil on the female genitals, you should use a water-based lubricant because if oil gets inside the vagina, it can cause irritation and infection.

Vulva Massage (also known as Yoni Massage)

Put the lube in your hands and rub your hands together before placing them on her vulva. Start by rubbing the lubricant on her inner thighs to tease her. Run your fingers through her pubic hair.

Flatten your hand and cup it over her entire vulva. If she is excited her labia majora (outer lips) will be engorged with blood. Do a patting or gentle slapping touch. This will draw more blood to her genitals and heighten the sensitivity to future touches. Trace the outline of her labia majora and labia minora. Gently pinch the folds of the labia between your forefinger and thumb. Run your lubricated fingers between the outer (majora) and inner (minora) lips to separate them.

Two-Lips

As you part her lips continue to caress them between your fingers. Rub them lightly in circular motions.

Use less pressure with the inner lips because they are more sensitive. Watch for her body language. Is she swollen? Open? Irritated? Red? Lubricated? Ask her for verbal feedback.

Clitoral Massage (also known as Pearl Massage)

Slide your fingers to either side of her pearl/clitoral hood and gently caress the pearl in circular motions. If you want to use your tongue for this, she will probably be delighted.

Every Story Deserves a Happy Ending

After massaging your partner's most intimate erogenous zones, it time for the Tantric finale as you cover your naked body in massage oil and climb on top of him or her massaging them with every part of your body, but not with your hands. You can slide your body up and down, side-to-side or grind your body in erotic circles into your partner's body.

"More important than the techniques is your own personal expression. More important than your own personal expression is the recipient's wishes."

– Dr. Kenneth Ray Stubbs

After a superbly erotic massage your partner negotiates how to conclude the experience. Maybe it's your turn to receive a Tantric massage or you both want to cuddle and then make love.

The Mind, Body and Energy Experience is a fantastic exploration all on its own that can take your relationship to a whole new level. Any growth in a relationship is dependent on trust and understanding and this journey is greatly enhanced by investing the time in learning to see your partner clearly. Personality similarities and differences are what create life's true romantic pleasures and knowing how to communicate effectively makes all the difference. Let's take a peek inside the science of personality and discuss the tools needed for an exciting Meeting of the Minds.

CHAPTER SIX
Meeting of the Minds

Relationships can sometimes feel like building a house in the middle of a storm. It takes an amazing amount of balance, courage, craftsmanship, concentration, and guesswork in order to build a safe haven while the winds of doubt and fear constantly threaten to blow away what you're trying to create. And the partner with whom you're sharing this experience brings along an entirely different set of tools that you must figure out how to use in order to complete the shared goal of safety. It can be scary, for sure, but if you figure out how to work together and utilize everything you both bring, you will not only create a safe shelter, but you will construct the home that will protect you throughout the adventure of life.

Our personalities are created by the building blocks of life experience: family guidance, education, community influence, and religious upbringing (or lack thereof). There are also internal

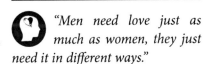 *"Men need love just as much as women, they just need it in different ways."*

– Dr. John Gray

architects at work that draw lines, which create our perceptions and responses, and each individual mind has its own blueprint. So how can we reconcile two minds with very different wiring into the same couple's dream house? And how can we learn to work together, especially during times when we seem to have nothing in common?

The answers are both simple and complicated. If you want to share electricity, you must first understand how each of you is wired.

Left Against Right

In 1981 Roger Sperry won a Nobel Prize for his breakthrough research that found that the brain divides activities into the left and right hemispheres, and the world hasn't been the same since. Countless studies, tests, books, presentations and discussions have happened since that revolutionary discovery that offered tremendous insight into the ways people interpret information differently.

We've all heard it said that the left-brain is associated with logic while the right is associated with creativity and intuition. According to respected psychiatrist and author, Dr. Iain McGilchrist, these claims are inaccurate. "One side isn't solely responsible for reason and logic and the other for emotion and imagination; we need both hemispheres for all of these functions."

Our left and right brains allow us to view reality with two different approaches. The brain is divided into four main lobes or regions: frontal (forethought and judgment), temporal (memory and mood stability), parietal (sensory processing and direction sense), and occipital lobes (visual processing). There are also important structures deep in the brain, such as the anterior cingulate gyrus (gear shifter), basal ganglia (anxiety and pleasure center), and deep limbic system (emotional center). The cerebral cortex manages rational functions and is divided into two hemispheres connected by a band of nerve fibers, known as the corpus callosum. These fibers relay messages back and forth between the two sides of the brain.

While both sides are utilized in nearly every activity, the left side of the brain manages the tools of language and works in a logical and sequential order. On the right side, visual information is processed, as are non-linear concepts like creativity.

The right brain is actually hugely responsible for the ideas that come to use in our dreams while we are sleeping. According to Jay Alfred, author of *Brains and Realities*, one of the founding fathers of quantum physics, Niels Bohr, came up with the concept of using a planetary system as the model for atoms. This concept led to the 'Bohr model' of atomic structure, which went on to win the Nobel Prize. This is a great example of the left and right brain processes working in tandem.

A 1999 study indicates that you may be able to know whether a person is predominantly left or right brained by observing the direction their eyes move. Canada's Robarts Research Institute studied conjugate lateral eye movements (CLEMS), which are involuntary eye movements to the left or right that can indicate a person's way of thinking. The results showed that people are predominantly left or right lookers and that 75% of their eye movements will be in one direction or the other. People with a tendency to glance to the right are more likely to be a left-brain, analytical type while creative, right-brain personalities will more often glance to the left.

Though some people have personalities that sit near the center of the scale, most have a dominant side. Just like being right-handed, the human brain is wired to lead with one side over the other. Knowing which side you and your partner tend toward can go a long way to diffusing conflicts when they arise.

Do you know your brain hemisphere preference? Take a look at these brief descriptions as presented by noted human consciousness pioneer and founder of The Monroe Institute, Robert Monroe. Does one list fit you better than the other?

Left Hemisphere Style RATIONAL	Right Hemisphere Style INTUITIVE
♥ Responds to verbal instructions	♥ Responds to visual instructions
♥ Looks for sequence	♥ Looks for patterns
♥ Looks at differences	♥ Looks at similarities
♥ Prefers to plan	♥ Prefers spontaneity
♥ Prefers established information	♥ Prefers elusive information
♥ Prefers talking and writing	♥ Prefers drawing and manipulating objects
♥ Prefers multiple choice tests	♥ Prefers open ended questions
♥ Controls feelings	♥ Free with feelings
♥ Sees cause and effect	♥ Sees correspondences

In her book *When Opposites Attract*, Rebecca Cutter outlines the different ways right-brain and left-brain people approach relationships. A left-brain thinker will start with the facts and then process through the emotions, while a right brain

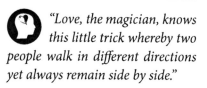

"Love, the magician, knows this little trick whereby two people walk in different directions yet always remain side by side."

– Hugh Prather

thinker will start with the emotions and then bring in the facts. Where two right brain people in a romantic relationship will use communication to feel more emotionally connected, two left-brain people will use communication to find a solution. In a relationship between opposite brains, the potential for conflict is obvious. How will two people with opposite approaches to life get along?

Common Complaints About A Left Brain Partner

1. Is emotionally unavailable to me.

2. Is preoccupied when we are together; obsessive.

3. Is not in the here and now; always in the past or future.

4. Is too inhibited; can't let go and play.

5. Is insensitive; too blunt.

Common Complaints About A Right Brain Partner

1. Gets too emotional when talking about problems.

2. Wants too much of my companionship.

3. Is too extroverted; draws attention.

4. Won't stay on one topic.

5. Does not take a logical approach to problem solving.

Two Rights Don't Make A Wrong

Does it help a relationship to have both individuals either left or right brained? Yes and no. In the case of right-brain couples, they benefit from the ability to communicate their thoughts and empathize with each other's emotions, so they give each other space when they need it and are touchy feely when they get the right signals from each other. Sounds too perfect to be true, right? Well, there's also a flip side. Two right brainers can be emotionally satisfied and creatively fulfilled, but they can also frustrate each other by frequently basing their decisions upon feelings rather than rationality.

One couple came to see me because they wanted me to help them create a mutual love contract to find out if they were compatible enough to get married. Bob and Christine were both artistic right-brained people who had been dating for almost a year and wanted to move in together. They eagerly collaborated on creating the love contract that included certain boundaries, such as no porn and no cheating. Clearly, they had the same deal breakers.

Then we addressed an area in the contract where they both wanted to adopt a dog and jointly care for it. They wanted to do it together as a prelude to becoming parents after marriage. A good idea, I told them, sharing my wish that more couples would practice taking care of animals before they had children. I told them to come back after they moved in together and had found the perfect pet, and to be sure to bring it to our next session. As an animal lover I encourage employees to bring their pets to work.

Six weeks later, they showed up with a chocolate colored Pomeranian who was a cute and happy bundle of fluff, weighing about ten pounds. "This is Bella," Christine said holding her like a baby, "She's about four years old and they think she was abandoned by a family who moved." Bob added, "Yes, and we just fell in love with her as soon as we saw her." I could definitely see the emotional connection they had with Bella.

"So, which one of you disciplines Bella?" I asked. Well, to cut a long story short, neither Bob nor Christine could bring themselves to reprimand Bella when she peed or pooped in their home. They also couldn't agree upon whether to feed Bella dog food or human food, so they gave her both and finally, they were too afraid to walk her in the park for fear that a bigger dog would attack her, so they always carried her.

Neither one of them wanted to be the 'bad guy' because they both wanted Bella's affection, but the lack of discipline was now impeding their own love life. Because they both had growing frustration about the inability to reprimand the dog, it was tainting how they felt in other aspects of their relationship. There was no doubt that they were giving Bella a lot of love and attention, but I cautioned them that without any rules or discipline this family was going to have problems.

I helped them to create some colorful problem solving charts to guide them in making decisions about Bella and other issues in their lives.

It included a Pro and Con list where they wrote down all of the good aspects in one column and all of the bad aspects in the other column. One of the pros was that they took turns initiating romantic dates and one of the cons was that Bella would interrupt their sex sessions, but they didn't have the heart to lock her out of the bedroom.

(If they had both been left-brainers, I would have told them to add a number to each of the pros and cons from 1 to 10 in order of importance so that they could measure the outcome quickly and effectively with a numeric score.)

The good news is that Bob and Christine used visual charts to determine what was best for Bella's wellbeing. By taking turns walking her, she got her exercise and they didn't compete for her attention. Then they applied this to all areas of their lives, from dinner party menus to their sex life.

The benefits of the visual love contract and the flow charts made it easy for them to measure and determine their level of satisfaction and progress in reaching their goals.

Two Lefts Can Be Right

Couples who both use their left-brain hemisphere primarily are less emotional, so less likely to argue. However, when a crisis does occur, this relationship can become strained by volatile emotions that neither one is accustomed to feeling.

My client Anita and her Indian boyfriend Vineet were both in the electronic engineering field, so their communication topics revolved around physics, math, computers and science, with no time for small talk or intimate conversation. They came to see me because they had heard that I lectured to couples in five cities in India. Anita initiated the session by saying that she wanted Vineet to make a commitment, as they had been dating for two years and her biological clock was ticking. Anita cited some statistics about how fertility declines for women from the age of 30 and she was already 29, so Vineet had to make up his mind one way or the other.

Vineet acknowledged her request by telling me that he had made a commitment to her by telling her that he loved her. The problem was that he wasn't ready for marriage or fatherhood until his career was more secure and he was a homeowner, both of which were taking longer than he had anticipated.

I asked Vineet about his parents and if their approval was also an issue. He shrugged unemotionally and said, "Parents today are more open-minded, even if they feel the woman is not right for their son."

That's when Anita's emotions came to the surface. "I knew it," she yelled. "Your mother insults me and you ignore it."

Vineet responded by saying quietly, "I've known my mother longer than I've known you, so rank has its privileges."

Anita had tears in her eyes but controlled herself as she turned to me and asked, "What is the solution?"

I asked them to share all of the things that they love about each other mentally, physically and emotionally, then to share the things that they want to improve in their relationship. Finally, I had them tell each other what they will not change in the relationship. The end result was that they both had deep feelings for each other, they both wanted to spend the rest of their lives together, but both wanted to be in control of every situation.

Vineet admitted that his mother would always come first, but Anita would be a close second. Anita admitted that she felt obligated to have a baby before she gets too old, and that she wanted to be married for at least six months before getting pregnant. She could accept that "rank has its privileges" and was willing to take a back seat to Vineet's mom. She was also willing to wait for marriage as long as they got engaged. Vineet agreed to the engagement by giving Anita his mother's diamond ring and both of them felt like they got their needs met.

My remedy for this relationship was for them to spend more quality time together sharing their emotions, so I gave them some love-work instead of homework. I told them to collaborate on creating a collage by cutting out various pictures that represent the life they want together. This helped them to communicate from the right side of their brain and prepare for a commitment resulting in a deeper level of intimacy, while resolving conflicts.

Opposites Attract & Detract

Many 'opposite' couples are excited by the differences in their world outlooks at first, but gradually those differences polarize the relationship. Janie and Roger came to me with such a dilemma. After five years of marriage, left-brained accountant Roger was becoming increasingly frustrated with right-brain music teacher Janie's attempts to engage him in the same conversations she had with her girlfriends, namely topics such as shopping, babies, spas and yoga classes. Janie thought it indicated a problem because he didn't share her interests. Because she was so passionately invested in these things, she interpreted his indifference toward these subjects as apathy toward her.

Only by coming to grips with their left vs. right differences and learning to accept the other's position as valid yet opposite, were they able to find a comfortable middle ground. Janie learned to save a majority of these conversations for her like-minded friends and only brought

"Both hemispheres of the brain are capable of some kind of awareness, but their methods of experiencing and expressing it are very different."

– Dr. Andrew Newberg

these subjects up with Roger when something required an action plan, such as her desire to remodel a portion of the garage into an art studio.

By becoming aware of how your messages are being perceived and making necessary adjustments to ensure proper communication, it becomes much easier to avoid misinterpretations that can lead to unnecessary arguments. This is especially important in the early stages of a relationship, before you have settled into a mutual understanding of how you both think and express emotion.

Whether partners are approaching things from the same hemisphere or from opposite sides of the fence, it's a great idea to strengthen the brain by challenging it with exercises that utilize opposing muscles. If your partner is of the 'opposite brain', these exercises can help you both as you reach for the middle. And if you both start from the left or right side, it's still unlikely that you will be on the exact same page, so these exercises will help inspire brain balance.

NEURO-CISE: RIGHT/LEFT BRAIN, SOLO

Here's a list of exercises showing which side of the brain will get the workout.

- ♥ Meditation (Right)
- ♥ Crossword puzzles (Left)
- ♥ Picturing a familiar face (Right)
- ♥ Calculations (Left)
- ♥ Writing with your non-dominant hand (Right)
- ♥ Writing with your dominant hand (Left)
- ♥ Fantasizing (Right)
- ♥ Organizing (Left)
- ♥ Repetitive movements (Right)
- ♥ Remembering a name (Left)
- ♥ Making love (Right)
- ♥ Analyzing a work of art (Left)
- ♥ Imagining how you would decorate a room (Right)
- ♥ Debating an issue (Left)

NEURO-CISE: BRAIN ACTIVATION, SOLO

If you wish to activate only the right side of the brain, you can close your right nostril by pressing your finger against it, and breathe only through the left nostril, thus activating the right side of the brain. You can also close the right nostril to activate the left side of your brain. This is a quick and easy way to tap into either brain hemisphere. If you wish to activate both sides of your brain, you can first close one nostril, breathe in and breathe out through your nose, then close the other nostril, breathe in and breathe out. This is an ancient yogi technique known as "Swara yoga" which leads to balance of both brain hemispheres.

NEURO-CISE: BRAIN ACTIVATION, DUO

You can activate sides of the brain by stimulating the opposite side of the body. The right brain awakens with a touch on the left side and vice versa, so a way to incorporate brain exercise with your physical intimacy is to take a tour of your partner's body, alternating from one side to the other. Consider taking this path for full body and full brain stimulation, and remember to take a pause between each side for the best effect:

- ♥ Temple
- ♥ Cheek
- ♥ Side of the mouth
- ♥ Ear
- ♥ Neck
- ♥ Shoulder
- ♥ Upper arm
- ♥ Forearm
- ♥ Hand
- ♥ Breast
- ♥ Ribcage
- ♥ Waist
- ♥ Outer thigh
- ♥ Inner thigh
- ♥ Buttock
- ♥ Calf
- ♥ Ankle
- ♥ Top of foot
- ♥ Bottom of foot
- ♥ Toes

The Extroversion Scale

Equally important to understanding where your partner fits on the left/right scale is to know where they sit on the scale of extroversion. Most people discuss the topic of introvert versus extrovert as if it is a black and white issue: a person is either one or the other. Like most things, however, the truth lies in the grey area. To this end, the term "ambivert" is slowly making its way into the mainstream. A term to describe someone who combines many elements of both extremes, an ambivert is actually the most common personality type.

One misconception about the difference between introverts and extroverts is that they are "antisocial" and "social," respectively. But it's much more instructive and accurate to examine how they restore their energy. In *The Introvert Advantage*, Psychologist Marti Olsen Laney uses this analogy to explain the difference: Introverts are like rechargeable batteries while extroverts are like solar panels. Introverts need to stop expending energy and rest in order to recharge while an extrovert sees this "down time" like being under a heavy cloud. Extroverts are recharged by the energy ("the sun") of other people while this social activity drains the power in an introvert.

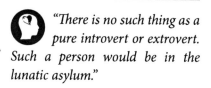

"There is no such thing as a pure introvert or extrovert. Such a person would be in the lunatic asylum."

– Dr. Carl G Jung

As it turns out, blood flow in the brain works differently for these two personality types as well. An extrovert's blood flows in a more direct path to the areas of the sensory processing centers for vision, sound, taste and touch, but curiously not to smell. This could be due to the fact that olfactory stimuli are closely linked with emotion, and if emotional processing were required to handle social interactions, then the path would be less direct, and therefore slowed down. On the other hand, an introvert's pathway is more complicated, with blood more easily flowing to the areas of the brain that handle the internal processes of memory, problem-solving, and planning.

Dopamine also plays a part in defining the differences between these two types. Extroverts have a low sensitivity to this 'feel good' neurotransmitter, yet they require large amounts of it so they are drawn to activities that trigger adrenaline which helps produce dopamine. Conversely, introverts are highly sensitive to dopamine and can quickly feel over-stimulated.

It's also important to note that being an introvert is not the same thing as being shy. As Dr. Laney defines the two, introversion is the propensity to tune into one's inner world while being shy is an extreme self-consciousness when around other people. While shyness may have genetic foundation, such as an overactive fear center, it is generally a learned behavior through life experience. Introverts enjoy social situations in controlled amounts while the same social gathering can instigate panic in a shy person.

NEURO-CISE: FOR THE INTROVERTED PARTNER, DUO

If your partner is an introvert, the best ways to love them is by being mindful of their needs:

1. Respect their desire for privacy.

2. Give them time to think. Instant answers don't come easy.

3. Don't interrupt them.

4. Allow them time to observe a public setting before making introductions.

5. Give them as much notice as possible if plans are going to change.

NEURO-CISE: FOR THE EXTROVERTED PARTNER, DUO

With extroverted partners, it's equally important to acknowledge and respect their needs:

1. Give them permission to "work a room."

2. Compliment them in front of others.

3. Give them options.

4. Encourage their adventurous spirit.

5. Thoughtfully surprise them.

An ambivert falls somewhere between these two extremes and most commonly balances near the middle. Comfortable in social situations but drained by them if they carry on too long, an ambivert keeps their energy in check by incorporating both socialness and solitude into their lives in equal measures.

A relationship between two people on different points of the extroversion scale can be challenging. An extrovert may struggle to understand why an introvert is not experiencing the same pleasure at a party, and an introvert may not comprehend why the extrovert doesn't want to spend a quiet day at home. However, there is much pleasure to be found in the dance of these opposing life approaches, once you recognize and respect them.

NEURO-CISE: INTROVERT EXPANSION, SOLO

If you're an introvert who would like to embrace some extrovert personality traits as a way to expand a social circle or romantic opportunities, here are some good ways to expand:

1. **Stop judging extroverts.** It can feel exhausting to imagine living a life as an extrovert when you focus on the extreme of the personality type but there's great happiness and comfort to be found in taking on the challenge of becoming more social.

2. **Envision your "perfect extrovert."** You don't need to be the center of attention in order to be more extroverted. Paint a picture in your mind of how you can comfortably test the boundaries of your extroversion and then tap into the emotional gratification that you will get from reaching your goals.

3. **Find a social group that works for you.** Join a club where you can utilize the things you enjoy doing on your own in a more social way, such as a book club, gym or singles community.

4. **Develop your social skills.** Talking to strangers is a learned habit that can feel exhausting or scary to an introvert. Remember to ask open ended questions and show genuine interest in the stories people have to share.

5. **Take your social life offline.** Make plans to have a real life face-to-face conversation with some of the friends you only ever socialize with via social media.

NEURO-CISE: EXTROVERT INTROSPECTION, SOLO

As an extrovert, the idea of trying to become more introverted may seem counter-productive to how the world tells us we should be, but that doesn't mean there isn't much to be learned by embracing the quiet time.

1. **Don't confuse introversion with shyness.** An introverted approach is not timid or bashful. It is simply quieter with more focus on ideas, observation, and imagination, all skills that can be used when you dive back into your more active social life.

2. **Explore your creativity.** One way to incorporate your extroversion into this exploration is to create art based on your 'louder life.' Keep a journal; write short stories about your adventures, sketch or paint.

3. **Appreciate solitary activities.** There will be times when solitude will be necessary for any number of reasons and learning how to see it as a gift instead of a curse will be helpful. Find things you enjoy that can be done on your own. Read, meditate, listen to music.

4. **Do it alone.** There are likely many things you usually do with other people that can be explored on our own. Go biking, hiking, do yoga or go to a movie.

5. **Self-nurture.** Many extroverts forget to take care of their personal needs because the focus is usually on a group. Carve out time for a spa treatment, massage, or even a nap.

Heart-To-Heart

Everybody has heard the old cliché that "opposites attract" and many would agree that it's true. Experiencing a different point of view can inspire us to see the world differently and with more empathy. But let's be honest, sometimes it seems that balancing these differences is like trying to push two opposing magnets together. You can get close, but the lack of compatibility makes a true connection impossible.

So what can we consider 'healthy' and 'unhealthy' opposites? In the long run of romance, which differences have the power to pull us together and which will push us apart? Are the most successful relationships built on similarities or differences? The answer may surprise you.

In one of the most extensive studies ever done about this topic, The University of Iowa found that the answer comes down to a single word: personality.

The Journal of Personality and Social Psychology published the findings of Psychologist Eva C. Klohnen, Ph.D., and graduate student Shanhong Luo, M.A., which showed that attitude, religion and values are the top reasons why couples get married, but similarities in personality remain key to a long, happy marriage. The authors state, "Once people are in a committed relationship, it is primarily personality similarity that influences marital happiness because being in a committed relationship entails regular interaction and requires extensive coordination in dealing with tasks, issues and problems of daily living. Whereas personality similarity is likely to facilitate this process, personality differences may result in more friction and conflict in daily life."

Building rapport between partners requires trust and an ability to see and accept the other as separate but equal. An important step in this process is first understanding our own self-image. The divide between our ideal selves (that we imagine we're projecting) and the actual image we project can cause a lot of strife.

NEURO-CISE: FACTS AND EMOTIONS, DUO

Any conversation between two people involves facts and emotions. Which do you focus on first? What about your partner? One way to clarify your natural inclination is by answering the following questions, making sure to share and discuss your separate answers:

In this relationship:

1. What expectations do I have of my partner?

2. What expectations do I have of myself?

3. What expectations do I believe my partner has of me?

4. What differences do we have that benefit our shared goal?

5. What differences do we have that cause me concern?

It's important to explore communication tools when things are good and comfortable because it's nearly impossible to remain objective and open minded when things

"Love without conversation is impossible."

– *Dr. Mortimer Adler*

are rough. Also, consider discussing things that are outside of the relationship in order to better understand how your partner thinks. For example, how a partner deals with work conflict gives some indication into how home conflicts will be approached. Are they direct or subtle? Do they talk more about what happened or how it felt? Is the response immediate or does it take a few days?

NEURO-CISE: CONVERSATION, DUO

When the time comes to have a serious conversation, it's important to be prepared. I'm not saying that every conversation needs to start with the lighting of a sacred candle while chanting a love mantra, but when it is an important discussion we must take the time to fully respect the needs of a serious conversation. Keep these ideas in mind:

♥ This is a discussion, not a lecture, so work to balance talking and listening.

♥ Make points or questions clear.

♥ Never assume to already know a person's point of view.

♥ Make a conscious decision to leave any old negative feelings about the situation in the past and start fresh with this interaction.

♥ Check body language to make sure it's sending the intended message. Head up. Shoulders relaxed. Arms and legs uncrossed.

♥ Practice active listening.

If you are unfamiliar with the term "active listening," it's a very simple technique that you are likely already using in other areas of your life without realizing it. It's when someone says something and the other person repeats what he or she heard in their own words. This gives the speaker the opportunity to tell the listener if what they heard is in fact what was meant. For example:

1st Person: "I get really worried when you are hours late and I have no idea where you are."

2nd Person: "So you're saying that if I'm going to be late I should give you a call, so that you won't worry?"

At that point, any clarification can be made in order to make sure both the intention and interpretation are correct.

Effective communication incorporates finding the right combination of words, body language, tone, speed and delivery. We must also keep in mind how the person we're speaking to is receiving the information. The majority of people speak to others in a manner that makes sense to their own heart-wiring, with the assumption that the intention will be clear, but this is not always the case.

Developed by Richard Bandler and John Grinder, Neuro-Linguistic Programming (NLP) breaks down three ways that information is sent and received: visual, kinesthetic, and auditory. Looking at the following overview, do you find yourself fitting one model more than the others? And can you confidently say which one fits your partner?

In neuro linguistic programming, the rule of thumb is to use a minimum of four body language cues to make deductions about a person's thoughts.

NEURO-CISE: NLP MODALITY, DUO

Given the hundreds of ways we can communicate, knowing the particulars of how your partner best receives information can go a long way to alleviating tension and creating harmony.

See. Look. Observe.
The "visual partner" wants to be admired for how good they look. They want to be seen as attractive, so tell them, "Your outfit looks great" or "Your hair looks really good that way." They want to see images, and they like to look at the person talking to them. They also enjoy someone who speaks with passion and has lots of expressive gestures.

Feel. Hold. Touch.
The "kinesthetic partner" is feeling-oriented. They like to be held, touched, stroked, and they like to hear what you are feeling and sensing when you are with them. They want to relish the emotional

feelings of words and favor slow, sensuous dialogue. Tell a kinesthetic person, "It feels so good to be with you" or "Your skin feels like silk."

Hear. Say. Listen.

The "auditory partner" is a good listener and likes the sound of words. They enjoy great detail and will often analyze what has been said. Tone of voice is important for an auditory person and the inflections used in a sentence can make the difference between ordinary

"On a metaphysical level, harmony between the brains means harmony and integration between our 'mental' bodies and our 'emotional' bodies."

– Jay Alfred

and extraordinary communication. Give an auditory person a lot of information about why you like being with them and what qualities you like most about them. Tell them "I like being with you because you have so much to say" or "Explain to me how that movie made you feel."

NEURO-CISE: THE 15 C'S, DUO

I created the 15 C's as "A Code for Creating a Confident & Charismatic Couple." Simply put, it's a friendly checklist of the elements that make up the strongest relationships that I've seen in my practice.

1. Courageousness

Any relationship takes courage. It takes courage to say the first "I'm sorry" and it takes guts to lower your guard enough to let a partner truly see who you are. It takes just as much bravery to make the commitment to stay in it for the long haul because there are going to be numerous challenges that test your strength, both as a couple and as an individual. These things might include:

♥ Saying "I love you" first.

♥ Asking for help.

♥ Admitting mistakes.

♥ Discussing family misconduct.

♥ Facing financial struggles.

♥ Confronting sexual needs.

Courage is often associated with gigantic acts of risk or valor such as having the audacity to sing in front of a crowd, the boldness to run for president, or the fearlessness to charge into a burning building to save people. These are obviously courageous and commendable actions that release dopamine (the fireworks of all chemicals), but there are smaller acts of courage that are no less admirable. Take some time to think about your life. The fact is, it is humanly impossible to reach adulthood without a few acts of courage. Thank your partner and tell them how you think they've been brave. We're taught not to be boastful, so hearing the words "I'm so impressed that you were able to do that" has a tremendous capacity to fill someone's day with gratitude and love.

2. Communication

We've talked a lot about communication throughout this book because it is the number one reason for both success and failure in a relationship. Remember that conversation is not always communication. Consider the three levels of communication: surface, intimate, and intuitive. Surface communication is everyday conversation: the weather, the work day, dinner plans, what's on TV, etc. Facts without emotional depth. With intimate communication, emotional issues, fears, and topics that require deep trust emerge. Intuitive communication is the ability to make thoughts and feelings clear without having to say a word. Your partnership has become part of your instinct, and you can read each other's needs clearly. Remember that left and right-brained people communicate differently, so be sure to approach your partner by using their predominant brain language and both of you will enjoy the lingering pleasure sensation of serotonin, the feel good chemical.

3. Chemistry

People think that you either have chemistry or you don't, and they are absolutely right! The limbic system, known as the seat of emotions, drives impulses and desires including sexual ones. So you can enhance your chemical attraction by doing the things you did when you first met, such as making out a lot or finding new erotic areas of mutual interest. Testosterone and estrogen, the male and female sexual hormones, will be triggered as you go deeper and share your fantasies. Expand your sexual horizons by making love in new positions and locations while flooding your body with feel-good endorphins. Chemistry can also be sparked with the element of surprise, so think outside the box!

4. Compatibility

Knowing where you're most compatible can go a long way to strengthen a relationship. Shared likes and interests create a lot of opportunity to connect through experience, discussion and the bonding chemical, oxytocin. Compatibility, closeness, romantic communication and behavior can raise oxytocin levels and lead to deeper intimacy.

Write down all the areas in your relationship where you already know you're compatible. It's a good reminder of the foundation you have in place. Then make a list of areas where you don't feel compatible. Together divide that list into two parts:

1. Areas where it's okay that you're not compatible and can agree to have different interests and pursuits.

2. Areas where you could find more compatibility with a little effort to share an interest.

5. Curiosity

One of the most powerful ways to keep a relationship fresh is to treat it with a constant sense of curiosity. Look at each other without history, if possible. See the person across the table from you, lying next to you in bed, as new. Be curious about his/her day. What did they do? Be curious about the parts of that person that you just don't know. Never pretend in a relationship that you really know the other person. Be curious about new and exciting facets of their personality, about what they really like. Always be curious about the next step in a relationship. Individually, and as a couple, keep curiosity as the heart center of your relationship and it will keep your brain firing up new neural pathways.

6. Contentment

Some people confuse contentment with boredom. There's nothing boring about feeling happy and safe. But it's important to maintain happiness through gratitude. Make a list of the things you're grateful for in your life with your partner. Tell each other on a regular basis how contented you are in your relationship. Call home from work for no reason at all except to tell your partner how great things are, and how much you love your life with your partner. Focus on the parts of your life that are working and have ease so that you have the strength to face challenges together. Give each other a quick fix of oxytocin with a heart-to-heart hug as a daily ritual and you might find that you both become addicted to the loving effect.

7. Collaboration

View everything that happens in your life as collaboration so that there is a sense of togetherness even when you're alone. This may cause the release of cortisol, the stress hormone, but the more that you can do together, the deeper the bond and the better you will feel. Make a list of gifts and talents that you bring to the relationship, and discuss how they could be purposefully mingled together. Make a wish list of the things that you've always wanted to do, either individually or together. How can you accomplish them through collaboration? The Journal Scientific American reports that collaboration is built into our genetic makeup and our brain function thrives around sharing, communicating and collaborating.

8. Commitment

Treat your commitment to each other like a sacred promise, not a hopeful dream. Review and renew any stated commitments you have in your life, like wedding vows, love agreements or specific plans. Celebrate anniversaries of when you first met, got engaged and married. Write a couple's mission statement! Make sure your commitments are still vital and relevant to how things may have evolved over time. Pair-bonder brains, including yours, are generally set up to attach to a mate. It happens mostly because of the neurochemical vasopressin, triggering lifelong attachment and commitment.

9. Copulation

Sex is a healthy part of an intimate bond and it should be treated with the same kind of attention given to other elements of the relationship. As time goes by and the comfort level grows, the hot and heavy sex that was once a big part of your connection may have moved to the back burner. That's fine and expected, but the back burner can generate just as much heat as the front one so be sure to turn it on every once in a while. And spice up the pot with some playful positions, experiment with different manual stimulations. Practice conscious copulation and don't "race to orgasm" but do increase the intimate connection that will lead you to a "braingasm" that lights up the entire brain.

10. Creativity

Seek out some interesting ways to keep the sparks alive. Decide on a list of creative projects that would be fun to do together, such as cooking, painting, dancing, writing a back-and-forth poem or story, taking an acting improv class, or redecorating one of the rooms of the house. Use your creativity for your date night. Instead of doing things that are passive, find things that you can do that are more active in nature: a romantic scavenger hunt, bubble bath followed by massage or a moonlight walk in the park or on a beach. Try looking at your sex life in a more creative fashion, too. Take turns being responsible for bringing creativity into all areas of your life, starting with your sex life. A study at Dartmouth College shows that the roots of creativity are found in eleven areas of the brain that make up the imagination "mental workplace," and that this playground stretches across the full brain-scape, making creative endeavors one of the best mental exercises available.

11. Consideration

Try doing one daily thing for each other that is purely an act of consideration, especially when your partner is sick. Make an appointment for them, take their clothes to the cleaners, get their car washed or just have their favorite drink ready when they come home. If your partner is not well, it's important to communicate that it's a temporary situation, and let them know you still find them desirable. If there is one thing daily that you can do for your partner, then you will feel more appreciated, and you will know that you are appreciating your partner. When you give love, you will receive love, and the ensuing oxytocin will help to maintain the bond, even if there is no sex.

12. Contribution

One of the most important aspects of being a couple is a sense of having a mission together. How can you as a couple contribute to other people's lives, to other people's projects? Find ways you can contribute to your neighborhood, to your community or charity, to your state, to your country. When a couple has the feeling that there is a strong sense of moral purpose at the core of their relationship, the couple has more reasons to make the relationship work, and there is much more of a grounded, spiritual nature. This is as important in the life of a couple as sexuality.

Paul Zak, founder of Claremont Graduate University's Center for Neuroeconomics studies found that oxytocin's ability to amplify feelings of trust, also spark generosity and contribution in a relationship. In fact, he found oxytocin to increase generosity by 80 percent. The subgenual cortex (which is activated by oxytocin) makes people feel good when they are doing something positive such as giving.

13. Compromise

Learning to compromise is one of the biggest lessons to be learned in a romantic relationship. Two people can't always have the same needs, opinions, and expectations, but they can become encoded by our memories, which are stored as a synthesis of different experiences and emotions. A relationship without challenge stops growing and becomes predictable, maybe even boring, like brain cells that stop growing. This can be especially true when partners having very different approaches to life and ways of processing of information. Your hearts might be in the right place, but if you're wires are crossed, then trouble ensues.

Communicating your needs will sustain the longevity of the relationship. You must address these issues from your point of view, not blaming the other person for what you do not get. You'll need to be honest enough to say what works for you and what does not, without blaming the other person. For example, if sex is the issue, you could say, "I know our sex life hasn't been the most exciting in the past few months, so I love your idea of trying to spice it up, but I'm not comfortable watching pornography. Perhaps we could go shopping for a fun sex toy to experiment with together." Or if lack of shared time together is the issue, you could say, "I know you hate sappy movies and I can't stand violent action films, but let's make a point to find a film we can both enjoy this weekend, because date night is really important to me." If you don't state what you want and offer a compromise, you can't expect things to magically work out.

14. Comedy

Speaking of magic, humor is a magical thing. True love takes hard work but if you don't find the time to laugh, what's the point of working so hard? Humor is a key element in any relationship, whether it is used as part of the initial flirtation

> *A well-developed sense of humor is the pole that adds balance to your steps as you walk the tightrope of life."*
>
> *– William Arthur Ward*

or as a stress diffuser many years into a long-term commitment. And we've all heard that laughter is the best medicine because when you laugh, your brain reacts by producing chemicals that make you feel happy.

Light-hearted humor, free of sarcasm or ridicule, can soothe conflicts by allowing you to address a concern without raised defenses or hurt feelings. The intent of humor should always be to communicate something positive and never to undermine, insult, or degrade your partner.

While the joys of laughter may be obvious, are you aware of its health benefits? Reduction of stress, stimulation of the immune system, a rise of the endorphins in the blood that work as painkillers, a decrease in systemic inflammation, and lowered blood pressure have all been linked to laughter. It's also healthy exercise. Dr. William Fry, a leading researcher in the psychology of laughter, says that 20 seconds of hearty laughter can quickly double the heart rate for up to five minutes, which is equal to the physical response to three minutes of vigorous rowing exercise.

"Laughter is the shortest distance between two people."

- Victor Borge, comedian, conductor and pianist

15. Celebration

Last, but definitely not least, is celebration. Couples who have a sense of celebration about their own lives and about their relationship don't just survive, they thrive. Celebration is a life attitude; it's not something you go out to do. Find ways to celebrate, and you will find more reasons to stay together. Not just anniversaries, but a beautiful day, a great meal, a fabulous date – these are all reasons to celebrate! Celebration implies play and a playful nature in a relationship will keep it fresh, young and exciting. Psychologists Dr. Wil Cunningham and Tabitha Kirkland at Ohio State University uncovered the effect while scanning brains of happy people and reported, "People with rose-tinted glasses are more responsive to positive things in the environment. But it's not at the expense of the negatives in life. They're not seeing the positives in everything, but they see the positives where they can find them."

Happy people respond more strongly to joyful objects and events in the world, their increased sensitivity helping to reinforce their happiness over time, and that's cause for celebration.

Mutual Love Agreement

Creating a love contract is a good exercise for any serious relationship. I have worked with several clients to create Mutual Love Agreements and they have proven incredibly beneficial for constructing and formalizing agreed upon relationship boundaries while clarifying needs and expectations. They work because both parties are able to express and negotiate their personal needs in a written format and hold each other accountable. It may sound like a lot of work, but it's actually a lot of fun.

NEURO-CISE: CREATE YOUR MUTUAL LOVE AGREEMENT, DUO

Start by working together to list as many relationship categories as you want to address. Examples: social, relationship, sexual, spiritual, family, financial, health, physical, vacation, career, parenting, pets and hobbies. This is a team effort. It must be created together so that neither partner feels coerced by the other.

Next, going section by section, outline your needs and wants for each category. Discuss options, ideas, and compromises until you have an agreed upon outline.

Finally, read and accept the partnership overview and then both sign and date it.

This shared commitment can also be used as a pre-marital agreement to help avoid conflict during the relationship.

Caution: It may not be admissible in a court of law unless it is approved by an attorney and notarized.

For the sake of creating a starting place for your own document, here is a sample agreement:

Dated: MM/DD/YY

By: _____ & _____

The party of the first part (herein referred to as 'name') being of sound mind agrees to the following with the party of the second part 'name.'

FULL DISCLOSURE: At the commencement of the Mutual Love Agreement each party agrees to fully disclose any current resentments, health issues, financial problems or relationship concerns.

DEFINITION OF RELATIONSHIP: Both parties mutually agree to use the following terminology in describing their relationship: committed, cohabitating and monogamous.

GOALS FOR OUR RELATIONSHIP: Total honesty, trust, respect and open communication.

SOCIAL: One night a week is designated to each party to go out separately with friends, business colleagues or family.

FINANCIAL: Parties will share a joint bank account plus maintain their own individual bank accounts. They will deposit their salary checks into the joint account which will be used to pay for living expenses including, but not limited to; rent, groceries, household items, utility bills, dining and vacations. Each party will keep the money they have accumulated before this agreement in their separate individual bank accounts. There will be no financial reimbursement from or to either party if this agreement is terminated.

SEXUAL: Parties will engage in sexual intercourse at least two (2) times a week, mutual oral sex at least three (3) times a week. Give each other a massage one (1) time a week. Watch porn once a month, but only together. Mutual masturbation at least one (1) time on weekends, unilateral masturbation, anytime.

BOUNDARIES: No hitting, no breaking things, no cheating, no bringing up old lovers, no shouting and no offensive name-calling.

SPIRITUAL: Each party respects the other's spiritual beliefs and does not attempt to persuade the other to change their faith.

PARENTING: When and if the parties do have children, they will be raised with no particular religion, but educated about all of them. Discipline will be mutually administered by both parties. The child or children will have both their mother's and father's last name, hyphenated with the mother's name first.

PETS: The parties will be mutually responsible for any pets, with a schedule agreed upon in advance for grooming, training, exercise and clean up. The parties agree to pay for complicated treatments that may arise during the pet's lifetime.

GROUNDS FOR TERMINATION: Any of the following will be grounds for immediate termination and final dissolution of said relationship: Physical violence, cheating with a man or woman and/or withholding sex for more than a month (unless for a medical reason.)

Agreed & Accepted

Dated: MM/DD/YY

By: _____ & _____

Side By Side

As you and your partner build the 'dream house' of your relationship, take advantage of all the astonishing insight gained from brain studies. Determine whether you're left or right-brained, auditory, kinesthetic or visual, and whether you're an extrovert or an introvert. Armed with this knowledge, relating to your partner becomes much easier, and arguments and negotiations become much more manageable.

Taking the time to fully understand the wiring of your partner's mind gives you great insight into how to stay strong in their heart. There will be times when it feels like work to see your partner clearly, but the payoff comes with a deeper, more 'in tune' connection.

There are many things that can derail a relationship that at one time appeared to be going full force in the right direction. Making an investment in your relationship by learning about each other, allowing for growth and change, and remaining passionate about keeping the connection strong helps ensure that the bumps in the road are merely rocks that can be moved to the side so the journey can continue. Regardless of what may come along, you must always feel like your partner is standing by your side, holding your hand.

As vital as it is to maintain a connection with each other, it's equally necessary to stay aware of your own needs. Read on, as we look at the tools necessary for taming the challenges of the Passion Assassins while working to create an even brighter path ahead.

CHAPTER SEVEN
Passion Assassins

"Love isn't practical. It isn't meant to be easy. It doesn't appear on command. It doesn't let you fall for whomever you'd like. It surfaces neither at the most opportune moment nor in the most convenient. It'll pair you with someone you might never have expected. It'll put you face to face with endless obstacles. But in the end, none of that will matter because it's how you overcome its obstacles that will define your love. It may not be practical, but love is ultimately the best thing that will ever happen to you." This anonymous quote sums up the purpose of this chapter, to help you recognize these endless obstacles so you can work to overcome them, and make your love stronger.

Like all things that are truly 'worth it', love isn't easy or stress-free. Each new challenge offers an opportunity to strengthen or destroy a couple's bond, and it takes real effort to choose the path that leads to success. The only difference between relationships that fly and ones that die is the way in which challenges are faced. Like a good workout, you can only get out of it what you put in. If you want to get strong, you have to do the heavy lifting, gain endurance, test your limits, and earn your sweat. A strong relationship requires the same elements as a strong body – a commitment to push forward when things get difficult, and the flexibility to adapt to new moves. If you don't stretch first, you could get hurt. And if you don't maintain the passion in your relationship, the bond will wither.

Defeating The Passion Assassins

So what kills passion? When I ask this question to my large group seminars, people often shout out things like, "Children!" "In-laws!" "Stress!" "Work!" Then I add things people might be too shy to call out: anger, hurt feelings, boredom, predictability, poor health, time constraints, fatigue, frustration, boredom, addictions, fear, family interference, rejection, unrealistic expectations, business problems, financial concerns, power struggles, lack of respect, lack of trust, lack of communication, overwork, resentments – it's a wonder any of us can maintain a healthy sex life!

It's overwhelming to think of all these obstacles working against you and your partner's happiness. Where do you start to tackle these issues? I like to begin by breaking down the enemy: distractions. By recognizing the internal and external distractions that tempt our attention on a daily basis, we have the potential to overcome them, and more fully experience all that gives us the most pleasure.

Let's start with external distractions. In his book, *Your Brain at Work,* Dr. David Rock states, "People everywhere seem to be experiencing an epidemic of overwhelm." We live in a world where we are constantly overrun with words, stories, images advertising, ideas, marketing, movies, television, music and news, and our technology is actually more advanced than human habit can fully comprehend. These distractions use a lot of what is a limited supply of attention that we have for each day. With each distraction that grabs your focus, your brain uses ketones, glucose, lactate, pyruvate and other energy substrates for neuronal efficiency. Because we are spreading these resources across several areas, each subsequent task makes you less effective than the last, especially in demanding circumstances, such as self-control and decision-making.

So how do these distractions affect our intimacy? What happens in the bedroom when we're checking our phones on the nightstand instead of sharing a kiss? And what habits can we put into place that pull us back to closeness?

My answer is both easy and bold. Turn off all devices of distraction. That's right; switch off your computer, the television, the radio, reading devices, and most importantly, your cell phone. Even turn the clock toward the wall so neither of you gets distracted by the time. This is an absolute necessity when trying to build, maintain or rediscover intimacy.

I can hear you all now with your excuses at the ready. *What if a big client calls? What if the kids need a ride? What if my stocks go up or down?* You may be interested to know that the reason your phone is so addictive is that when someone texts or calls you, it triggers a dopamine release, sending signals to the reward center of your brain. Like the pull of an addictive drug, it's too tempting not to respond. But ask yourself this: Do you want to be a drug addict or do you want a successful relationship? You can call your client back, you can pre-arrange your children's schedules - it's a matter of priority. And when you prioritize your relationship, you get positive results.

Keeping with the bedroom scenario for now, let's talk about the environment of your bedroom, which can profoundly affect both men and women. For example, if you have a messy bedroom, what kinds of distractions might prevent you from being intimate? Our world is filled with mood triggers that we may fail to notice. A messy bedroom that has dirty laundry, leftover food, and scattered shoes or kids toys activates the stress hormone cortisol, and can lead to anxiety and even sexual dysfunction, while a clean, distraction-free room can inspire the brain's release of serotonin. An increase in this feel-good" neurotransmitter makes us feel happier and calmer.

Wired with a caretaker's brain, many women cannot fully relax in a messy bedroom because they feel a responsibility to make everything perfect. Yale professor Amy Arnsten goes so far as to call this need for perfection the "Goldilocks of the Brain." In order to function at an optimal level, the pre-frontal cortex, needs to have everything "just right." While this applies to both sexes, it is more often that untidy surroundings will distress women. Comfortable surroundings allow for the release of oxytocin and the emotional attachment it inspires. Oxytocin lowers a woman's stress and, for it to make an entrance, everything needs to be just right.

Once you have created a non-stressful environment by removing as many distractions as possible, you can fully focus on you and your partner's pleasure, spiking his testosterone and her estrogen, two major players in sex drive. Remember to turn the clock around so that it doesn't distract from focusing on intimacy, as some people unconsciously hurry lovemaking fearing they are taking too long to climax. This is especially true for women.

Other external distractions involve third parties, like pets, children, in-laws, work deadlines and personal schedules. These issues need to be dealt with one by one, with a goal of carving out time for intimacy. Put your dog or cat out before getting intimate, as they will forgive you a lot easier than your partner. Tell the kids that you are going to have some private time and lock your bedroom door so they can't come in to surprise you in the middle of your orgasm. If your mother-in-law has a tendency to show up unannounced, give her specific days and times that are off limits and tell her to call before coming over. As a couple, you are entitled to having strict rules that will enable you to have more quality time together.

Unfortunately, internal distractions don't have such an easy, tangible fix. You can't just switch off your brain. We have as many as 7,000 thoughts per day, many of them variations or repeats of the same insecurities, questions, doubts, and fears that forever cycle around our minds. As Dr. Rock explains, "If you were to look at the electrical activity even in a resting brain, it would look like planet earth from space with electrical storms lighting up different regions several times a second."

When it comes to profound internal distractions like resentment, lack of trust or frustration with your partner, it's imperative that you work through your issues together. One couple I counseled was trying to get over an act of infidelity. He had cheated and she was devastated, but attempting to move on and re-establish trust. Their sex life was hugely affected by the transgression because she could not stop thinking about his attraction to another person, which made her feel unwanted and sexually unattractive. One way to move beyond this feeling of inadequacy is to be bold and focus on your pleasure as you state your desires, so your partner learns how to please you physically. Do tell him what you need, for example, "I need you to go down on me until I come, then I want you inside me." This will help reignite the bonding chemicals, as you are getting your sexual needs met and he is aroused by sexual confidence.

Directing all of your focus on a single mission can silence internal distractions because you are not leaving room for multiple ideas to pull your attention. For the woman

"We must act out passion before we can feel it."

– Jean-Paul Sartre

above, by making her own orgasm the only goal, she leaves no space for insecurities and the pain of her husband's infidelity to penetrate her mind. Even when we're sitting still, we have a tendency to be multi-tasking, if only in our thoughts, so learning to create a single, clear mindful path is a necessary step in building a great life and glorious love.

NEURO-CISE: DISTRACTION EXTRACTION, SOLO

We don't often realize how many distractions we're juggling because they have simply become a part of our everyday life. Here are two simple ways to build awareness of the distractions you face:

1. **Look around for 10 minutes.** Sit comfortably in an area of your home where you spend a great deal of conscious time, the living room perhaps, and dedicate 10 minutes to

observing your surroundings. Does the cat jump on your lap? Does the phone ring? Kids shout? Is the television on? Are your partner's shoes in the middle of the floor?

2. **Look at nothing for 10 minutes.** Locate a blank wall in your home and pull up a chair and just look at the blankness for 10 minutes. While this exercise may begin with you analyzing the wall - the paint, the crack that needs fixing – you will likely find that it quickly evolves into an internal monologue of the various thoughts, questions, desires, dreams, mistakes, wonders and ideas that create the scope of interior distractions.

Combining these two exercises helps build awareness of how many hurdles are being jumped in a day. Many times simply acknowledging something helps reduce its need for attention. At the very least, you will gain a clearer picture of where your focus is being pulled.

NEURO-CISE: DISTRACTION EXTRACTION, DUO

Many times when partners come together for intimacy, which may or may not lead to sex, they each bring with them a gaggle of invisible thought balloons that hover around and between them, making the attempt to connect feel like "one more thing that needs my attention." Try this as a way to shoo those mind distractions away:

1. Reduce as many external distractions as possible. If you want to incorporate music, use something instrumental versus something with a singer because consciously or subconsciously we will at least partially be paying attention to the lyrics.

2. Stand or sit facing each other and take a few deep breaths with eye contact.

3. Each of you then rubs your own hands together to create a bit of warmth.

4. Raise your hands and place them palm-to-palm against your partner's.

5. Take a deep breath simply feeling the warm energy in your partner's hand.

6. Slowly rotate one of your joined hands in a small circle and silently acknowledge the most pressing mental distractions that come to mind.

7. Treat these distractions as if they were demanding children and silently ask them to wait their turn and to come back in an hour.

8. Move back and forth for a few moments between your joined hands, each time making a small circle and asking a distraction to come back in an hour.

While doing this exercise you will likely find that your focus moves between the distractions you're trying to release and the feel of your partner's hand and the look on their face as they do the same. You may begin to share the things you're thinking about, you might giggle or smile, or you could discover a simple pleasure in the connection as you settle into the moment together. Regardless of the response, the message being shared with your partner is "In this moment, I am working to give you my full focus" and, even in silence, that speaks volumes.

The Tall Tale of Multi-Tasking

The needs of a relationship are often lumped in with a variety of life's demands, and we include those duties as part of our attempt at multi-tasking. We have serious conversations while watching television. We respond to romantic emails while working on a financial

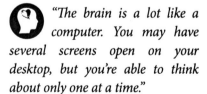

"The brain is a lot like a computer. You may have several screens open on your desktop, but you're able to think about only one at a time."

- William Stixrud, PhD

spreadsheet. We plan our anniversary celebration on the phone while racing between meetings.

The reality is, it is physically impossible for the brain to multi-task. Our minds can only efficiently process a single thought, action or task at a time. You are not asking your brain to do many things at once as much as you are asking your brain to quickly shift focus from one thing to another, an action known as "spotlighting." Though you may think that jumping from work to home to family to friends to kids to spouse and back to work is productive, attempting to multi-task actually takes a negative toll. According to Margaret Moore, co-author of *Organize Your Mind, Organize Your Life*, some of these harmful side effects may include:

♥ An inability to focus well on any one activity.

♥ Feeling rushed all the time.

♥ Feeling unproductive when only doing one thing.

♥ Impatience and lack of empathy for others who are often seen as getting in the way.

While it may seem that the concept of multi-tasking increases productivity because several things are moving forward simultaneously, the opposite effect may actually be taking place. Stanford researcher Clifford Nass had a theory that people who considered themselves successful multitaskers had simply honed their skills of spotlighting (switching focus from one task to another) and would thereby excel in filtering information and maintain a high working memory. This proved to be completely untrue. "Single-taskers" were better at defining irrelevant information and found it easier to switch between subjects.

To be most successful, we need to strive for singleness and to do ONE task at a time. This includes the needs of our romantic relationships. Time must be taken every day to give 100% of our focus to our partner and the life we share.

NEURO-CISE: FOCUSING, SOLO

A good starting point for finding focus is a good, old-fashioned To Do list. Part of the reason we mentally multi-task is because we are trying to juggle and remember everything we need to get done. The simple act of getting it down on paper alleviates the stress of forgetting something.

Prioritize the list and then give full focus to each item. If there are several things that need to get done in a day, one technique to consider is The Pomodoro Technique®. This simple method breaks up activities into 20-minute segments. Using a timer, select a task that needs to get done and then dedicate 20 solid, uninterrupted minutes to getting the job done. Silence your phone, close your email notifications, turn off the television and put 100% of your focus on the task at hand. When the timer goes off, take a short break to rest your eyes and mind, and then reset the alarm for another 20-minute session dedicated to a different task.

It sounds simple and you may not believe that 20 minutes is enough time to accomplish much of anything but, if you try it, I believe you'll be shocked at how much you get done in these bursts of laser focus.

NEURO-CISE: FOCUSING, DUO

If you're going to insist on multi-tasking, do your best to reduce it to two things: enhancing your relationship and exploring an activity.

Relationship-building (and maintenance) can itself feel like a multi-tasking activity but the simple act of doing something together can make this work easy and fun. Consider these three flirtatious options for bringing a scattered mind into focus:

♥ **Get naked.** How easy is that? When you're at home with your partner, strip down and go about your usual activities. This is an especially powerful trick when trying to get a man to pay attention. More responsive to visual stimuli than women, the male brain will force mental focus to be given to your exposed body.

♥ **Blindfolded phone sex**. By removing all of the senses other than sound, full focus is placed on the words, ideas, desires and fantasies being shared.

♥ **Sensation play**. Using extreme temperatures on the body pulls all concentration to the physical sensation. An ice cube tapped on various regions of the body creates a pinpoint awareness of anticipation and the excitement of the dance between pleasure and pain. More adventurous partners might explore the opposite extreme of heat by dripping paraffin candle wax on one another, though this takes serious trust, consideration and caution.

Mismatched Sex Drive

Throughout the course of a relationship, there will likely be times when libidos simply don't match for a variety of reasons, most of which have nothing to do with the actual intimate relationship. Stress, personal

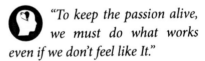

"To keep the passion alive, we must do what works even if we don't feel like It."

– Dr. John Gray

health, emotional wellbeing, exhaustion, work anxiety, and times of great challenge and/or change can have adverse effects. For some, these issues will cause an increase in sexual desire as a way to escape. Other people will find their feelings of lust decrease dramatically while facing these challenges. This imbalance can cause a lot of strife if it isn't understood and respected.

There really isn't any way to define a "normal" sex drive. There are many couples that have sex one or two times a month, and are completely satisfied. The only time there could be cause for concern, is when a couple's sex drives are not parallel.

There are several reasons why a couple may not be in the mood at the same time. It could be physical: too tired, a medical condition, or certain medications affecting arousal. It could be emotional: too stressed, feeling emotionally deprived by a partner, or unresolved issues. It could also be just plain boredom. Look, it's no secret that a relationship can get stale after a while. Like anything else, if we don't put effort into creating a great sex life, it could all be over once the "honeymoon phase" ends; you know, the first 2-3 months (if you're lucky) in the beginning when attraction seems effortless.

According to a 2002 study by the highly respected National Opinion Research Center at the University of Chicago, married couples say they have sex 68.5 times a year, or slightly more than once a week. That may not sound like a lot, but contrary to popular belief, married people have 6.9 more sexual encounters a year than people who have never been married. After all, you can't underestimate the value of having a willing partner conveniently located in bed next to you!

If one member of the couple is attempting initiation, and the other constantly refuses, the person with the lower sex drive can tend to feel barraged and possibly even harassed. The one who is feeling the desire more often can feel neglected, unattractive, and unloved. Arguments occur, and the sex slowly slips away. When the sex slips away, so does the casual affection like kissing, caressing, hand holding, laughing at each other's jokes, and the playfulness that comes with intimacy.

NEURO-CISE: SEX DRIVE, DUO

It all comes down to negotiation, communication, and making the decision to be receptive to your partner's advances. Easier said than done, but there is hope!

Step 1: Determine if both of you are being realistic or if one of you is just plain greedy.

Step 2: Define the problem by finding out if your partner is okay. Show concern and find out the main cause for the lack of desire. Don't pressure or blame your partner, be supportive, listen and acknowledge the problem. Then ask what you can do to help make them feel better.

Step 3: Compromise so that you both get your needs met. Here are some added solutions for aligning your sex drives:

- ♥ Make a "date night." Pick a day and time and fully enjoy each other by appreciating the whole person without demanding or expecting a performance. Take turns initiating and organizing the date.

- ♥ Give one another a sensual massage, caressing every inch, focusing on the non-sexual erogenous zones (back of the neck, navel, hips, thighs, behind the knees).

- ♥ Bathe together. Take turns washing each other's backs, arms, legs, and stomach. Soap up and rinse down from head to toe.

- ♥ Set the mood. Take your time and allow your partner to get in the mood; whisper compliments in each other's ear at dinner; tell you partner what you'd like to do to him/her later that night.

- ♥ Make intimacy a priority by putting as much time and energy into it as you do for jobs and children.

The fact is, you can't just sit around waiting to get in the mood. The key is foreplay. Not just what you do two minutes before you want to have sex; it's about setting the mood whenever you're around your partner. This can easily be done with a scratch of a back, an unpredictable kiss or a simple compliment. Games are also excellent mood setters. I created my Tantric Lover's Game to get couples on the same page and allow them to experience new exciting techniques that can take their relationship to a whole new level of intimacy.

Remember, never make someone else responsible for your sex drive. While you can ask for support, it's up to you to make the decision to get to where you would like to be sexually.

Willpower Reimagined

Focus takes willpower and meditation is good for both. Don't skim this section! There is good news at the end for those of you who insist you're bad at meditation.

Regardless of the available scientific research from Harvard University where studies show that 12 minutes per day for eight weeks of meditation results in significant improvements to brain function (among the many, many, MANY other benefits), it is an activity some simply can't comprehend. "How am I supposed to sit still and think of nothing? If I'm thinking of nothing ... isn't that thinking about something?" Well, here's a secret: trying and failing to meditate actually trains your brain to be good at having willpower! Did you hear that? BEING BAD AT MEDITATION IS A KEY TO GETTING GOOD AT WILLPOWER. Woo hoo!

Drs. Ruth Buczynski and Kelly McGonigal presented a webinar session on this topic for The National Institute for the Clinical Application of Behavioral Medicine (NICABM). Author of *The Willpower Instinct,* Dr. McGonigal argues that there are actually three kinds of powers we need in order to accomplish difficult tasks. She calls these I Will Power, I Won't Power, and I Want Power.

"I Won't Power" is actually what most people think of when defining willpower: the ability to resist temptation. "No dessert for me tonight" or "Thank you, but I quit smoking."

"I Will Power" is finding the strength to go through with something that feels uncomfortable. "This boring report is due tomorrow but I'm determined to finish it" or "I probably don't need to go but I'm going to follow through with this doctor's appointment anyway."

"I Want Power" is the one most people never consider. It takes into consideration the big picture vision of a desired life. This power is at the deepest core of the previous two. "I want my marriage to work so I will ignore your flirtations" or "We want to buy a house this year so we'll have to trade a vacation for a stay-cation."

Combining these three elements creates the full world of willpower, which resides in the brain as a collection of zones in and just behind the eyes in the prefrontal cortex. It is here that you store the list of things you want, shared between the

"These three skills—self-awareness, self-care, and remembering what matter most—are the foundation for self-control."

– Dr. Kelly McGonigal

two sides of the prefrontal cortex. The right side manages the desires of the "I Won't Power" by controlling attention and behaviors, while "I Will Power" lives more in the left side where motivation keeps you moving toward something regardless of stress or temptation.

Okay, okay ... so what's this business about weak meditation building strong willpower? Well, at its most basic, meditation is little more than concentration, and this exercise takes the ultimate willpower, especially for those who struggle to sit still with a clear mind. You basically use the same tools for different goals, which Dr. McGonigal describes as "having a goal, paying attention to what is happening in your mind and body and what's moving away from that goal, and then coming back to it."

NEURO-CISES: WILLPOWER, SOLO

To strengthen the muscles of willpower, perform the following five-minute exercise:

1. Sit still and focus all of your attention on your breathing.

2. Notice when your mind starts to wander, because it will and that is okay.

3. Take note of where your thoughts take you, accept these ideas with gratitude and then return your focus to your breathing.

4. Make a five-minute commitment to stillness and breathing but allow your mind to wander, knowing you will simply pull your thoughts back to your breath.

Acknowledging that your mind can tempt you to do other things, to put focus elsewhere, but maintaining a commitment to return to the goal of listening to your breath strengthens the subconscious understanding of your capacity for willpower.

Loosen The Grip Of Stress

In these demanding times, stress is inevitable but not unmanageable. In fact, managing stress is an absolute requirement for health and safety.

The area of the brain that responds to stress is the limbic system, often referred to as the "emotional brain." Whenever

> *"Meditation is not a way of making your mind quiet. It is a way of entering into the quiet that is already there - buried under the 50,000 thoughts the average person thinks every day."*
>
> *– Dr. Deepak Chopra*

you perceive a threat, whether real or imagined, this area of the brain responds through the sympathetic nervous system which, in turn, releases a series of hormones, including adrenaline, that increase breathing, heart-rate, and blood pressure. This sends oxygen-rich blood to the brain and to the muscles required for a fight or flight response. Your senses heighten, your memory sharpens, and you are less sensitive to pain. None of these side effects seem that bad, right? In fact, who wouldn't want to be that alert more often?

The problem is, other functions shut down during a perceived emergency because they are deemed unnecessary. Growth, reproduction, and the immune system are put on hold while blood flow to the skin is reduced. This is why sexual dysfunction, increased illness, and skin ailments are all negative side effects of long-term stress.

It should be noted that the goal is stress management, not stress elimination, as appropriate stress is a healthy part of life. Norepinephrine is also released during times of stress and this neurotransmitter aids in the creation of new memories, improves mood, and inspires creative thinking. It's a fine balance though, as the release of excessive stress hormones such as cortisol has a negative effect on the brain, most notably on memory. Cortisol scrambles the messages traveling between brain cells, thereby suppressing the ability to think or retrieve memories.

Learning stress management techniques can assist with every aspect of your life because anxiety carries with you even when you're outside of the stressful situation. For instance, a tense and worrisome day job

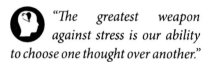

"The greatest weapon against stress is our ability to choose one thought over another."

– William James

will affect your state of mind outside of the office as well. The first step in alleviating stress is to clearly analyze the cause of your anguish. To say "my relationship with my in-laws is stressful" is not enough. Even "my father-in-law's expectations are too high" isn't taking the analysis far enough. You must keep asking yourself why until the answer moves from the external to the internal. Unlike inflicted physical pain, which you cannot control, stress is an emotional reaction to a situation, and our emotions are either conscious or unconscious choices. To say stress is a choice may be a bold statement, but it's also an empowering one because it means a less stressful life is something you can create.

The Mayo Clinic is widely credited with outlining the Four A's of Stress Release: Avoid, Alert, Accept, and Adapt. Each of these concepts offers genuine insight into relieving life's stress, from the most basic to the most severe.

Avoid

Many stressful situations can simply be avoided when we become aware of the fact that this option actually exists. Sometimes we find ourselves in tense circumstances simply because we didn't want to hurt someone's feelings or felt obligated to do something that we knew to be troublesome. Much can be gained by learning to take control of your surroundings. Avoid people and tasks that make things challenging. Sometimes this isn't possible but many times it is. Learn to say no to experiences you know will be stressful for you. So if your boss asks you to feed his or her cat while they are out of town and you are allergic to cats, instead of trying to please your boss, be honest by saying, "I would love to help you out, but my allergy to dander would make me sick for days so I couldn't work on that project you need me to finish." You may feel guilty about turning down the request, but the good news is that your boss will never ask you again and will be happy with your honesty that results in you being more productive.

Another way to avoid stress is to take an honest look at your To-Do list. Most of us have it in our heads that at least 90% of the list is urgent, so we constantly feel overwhelmed to get it done. In reality, the absolute priority items may make up as little as 10% of the list. The rest can wait, be delegated, or maybe even just crossed off.

Alter

Another way to overhaul the stress in your life is to make changes in how you approach demanding circumstances. Instead of silently seething about the behavior of others, respectfully ask them to change what they're doing. If you know that the reason you find it stressful to have friends over for dinner is that your partner makes jokes about your cooking, ask them kindly to stop. You have to communicate your feelings openly, but remember to use "I" statements, as in, "I feel disrespected when you make fun of my meatloaf in front of our friends." Time management is another way to alter things to become less stressful. In the case of our dinner party with friends, instead of stopping at the market on the way home to hastily throw together a four-course meal in two hours, what prep work might be able to be started the night before? And if a guest offers to bring a dish or dessert, why not let them? Stating limitations is also a great way to alter a possibly stressful situation. If your partner calls midday and asks if you can host dinner that evening, it's well within your right to say, "I don't have time to make a full dinner but I am happy to pick up pizza on the way home from work and then I can throw together a salad from what we already have in the refrigerator."

Accept

The third A in the list may actually be the hardest one to, well, accept. Sometimes there is no choice in the matter and we must simply accept a difficult situation. It's stressful to try to change something that is unchangeable, and in these unique situations, it is only through acceptance that the stress is released. Talk about it with someone - your partner, a friend, a minister or a counselor. Expressing frustration can sometimes alleviate its power over you, even if the situation can't change. For example, a partner's illness may challenge us to let go since we can't fix it. Men in particular struggle with this since they are wired to be "fixers", who may mistake acceptance for defeat.

A father may become stressed when his daughter doesn't make the basketball team and try to work every angle to get her a spot, including working with her extensively on getting better and begging the coach to give her a chance. Not only is he creating a stressful situation for himself but also everyone else around him. By accepting that she isn't a good enough player for the team, he is able to put that focus on the skills where she does excel, which not only reduces his stress but also enhances her self-esteem.

Forgiveness also plays a big part in acceptance, and sometimes the person who most needs to be forgiven is ourselves. Guilty feelings about anger, disappointment, and grief are often at the root of situational stress, and those feelings must be acknowledged and forgiven before the stress can be released.

Adapt

The final A is for adapting to new situations instead of holding onto the way things were. Changing expectations is an excellent way to alleviate stress. For example, children teach us how to adapt. As much as we may plan for their arrival and expect a particular series of events to unfold, they still turn our lives upside down, in ways we could never have imagined, but we adapt. We learn to take naps whenever we can, we discover how to shower with one eye on a toddler and we find parenting groups to discuss the new stresses in our lives. We focus on the joy of the baby's first steps, not the drudgery of cleaning dirty diapers. We find ways to make our new situation feel good.

I like the expression "God laughs when we make plans," because it speaks to the necessity for flexibility and adaptation. No matter how hard we try, we can never know what will happen next in our lives, and forcing a particular agenda can often block a bigger success in another direction. Let's face it, without adaptation; the human race would have died off long ago.

If you're having difficulty adapting to a new situation, try this: Reframe the issue so that oppositions are seen as opportunities. Adopt a mantra that makes you feel powerful and share it with your partner. "I can handle this" takes on much more strength when it becomes "We can handle this." You have two choices – you can feel sorry for yourself and push your partner away, or rebound from the unexpected challenge and team up with your partner to make a better life.

Regardless of which of the A's you apply to your situation, always remember to keep the big picture in mind. Ask yourself, "In five years, will this matter? Will I even remember this particular stressor?" The answer is quite often "no." And if you think it's at all possible that today's story might be funny tomorrow, why put the laugh on hold? Nothing releases the pressure of stress like laughter.

NEURO-CISE: PROGRESSIVE MUSCLE RELAXATION, SOLO

Progressive muscle relaxation is a great way to reduce stress by concentrating on physical sensations. This is done by slowly tensing and then relaxing the muscle groups. By both creating the tension as well as the relief, it helps the brain retain a sense of control that may feel lost during a stressful situation.

♥ Begin by finding a comfortable place to sit or lay down where you won't be interrupted for at least five minutes. Remove your shoes, if that helps you relax.

♥ Starting with your toes, clench the muscles and hold the tension for five seconds.

♥ Release and relax for 30 seconds.

♥ Repeat this process with all of the muscle groups, slowly moving up the body to the legs, pelvis, buttocks, stomach, hands, chest, shoulder, neck, and jaw, tensing each for five seconds and then relaxing for 30 seconds before moving to the next set of muscles.

Raising Self Esteem

Many of the challenges that interfere with passion have their root in issues of self-esteem. We try to manage situations in which we feel trapped, we confuse 'people pleasing' with 'self-defeating', and suppress our own needs in order to be perceived as generous rather than selfish. But most of us are in no danger of being selfish and genuinely need to examine our self-concepts.

Before you can begin to improve your self-image you must first believe that you deserve it, and then conceive it and you will achieve it. Change doesn't always happen quickly or easily, but it can and will happen if you really want it to.

You have the power to improve your self-esteem, but the first step is to accept and take full responsibility for your own power.

The second and most important step is to have a positive attitude. A positive attitude is the latent power you have within you, to bring about what you want. It is your own personal "happy face" designed just for you. A

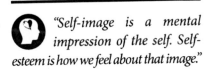

"Self-image is a mental impression of the self. Self-esteem is how we feel about that image."

– Rebecca Cutter

positive attitude is your ally; it is on your side no matter what. Your attitude is your response to the events in your life, so be careful not to overreact automatically. You cannot change other people, but you can change the way you view them, and they will most likely respond to your positivity with more positivity.

The fact is that you have thousands of thoughts a day and you have the choice about what those thoughts are going to be, whether they are positive or negative. Those thoughts are what act on the brain to release the neurotransmitters that affect our mood and health.

You also have the choice to select an attitude that works with you rather than against you. That choice can make or break your day, week, month, even your life. A positive attitude is more valuable than education, talent, wealth, and triumph. It can turn a failure into a success because if you react with a positive attitude, then things can only get better. Life continuously produces your feelings concerning it! Examine what choices you have been making for yourself unconsciously and make a conscious effort to focus on the positive side. Your positive attitude will be contagious, especially if you make the time to personally thank everyone who is helpful, courteous, professional or good to you.

NEURO-CISE: POSITIVE ATTITUDE, SOLO

To maintain a positive attitude you must practice, because it not only makes perfect, it perfects what it makes.

1. Write down as many causes as you can for feelings of poor self-image. It could be when someone said something unkind to you, or a time when you felt taken advantage of, or an overall feeling of weakness or insignificance.

2. Stop criticizing yourself and replace negative feelings with appreciative ones.

3. List all of your accomplishments, big and small.

4. Identify all of the unique qualities that you have to bring to a friendship. Write them all down and look at them regularly.

5. Practice self-love by treating yourself as a valuable person. Pamper yourself every single day by doing something that makes you feel happy.

6. Turn on your positive attitude switch and ask yourself, with confidence. "What personality and character would I need to possess to have the life I really want?"

7. Decide how you would like to be perceived, then visualize yourself in a situation where you are standing tall, your head is held high, and you have the persona that you want. Faking it at first is all right because soon you and your new image will be as one.

8. Write down all the emotions you want to feel as people react to you in a positive way.

9. What would you like your body image to express to others? Example: Healthy, sexy, sophisticated, strong, etc. Say the answers out loud and then write them down.

10. Look at yourself from your feet to the top of your head, preferably naked. Pause at each part of your body. Don't move upward until you identify something positive and say it out loud. Example: "My toes are perfectly shaped," or "I love my shoulders."

11. Say 3 affirmations before you start your day every day. Examples: "I am worthy of being loved" or "I'm a great catch for someone" or "I love and accept myself." Repeat these affirmations throughout the day, 10 times each.

12. Imagine how it would feel if all your dreams came true. Now tap into those powerful emotions and carry this feeling with you throughout each day.

Negotiating Compromises

Negotiating in relationships is the same as negotiating in business. In both cases, the goal is to make yourself and your partner happy, and in both cases, communicating needs will sustain the longevity of the partnership. It is also true that employees with good relationships at home can increase profitability at work. Statistics point to the price of divorce and the impact it has on corporate America, with an estimated $30 billion in federal and state costs to taxpayers. Failing relationships also cause decreased productivity and unhappy employees who quite often develop serious health issues. Learning to compromise and get your needs met at the same time is paramount to a good working situation and a great relationship.

Disagreements are bound to happen. Two people can't always have the same needs, opinions, and expectations. A relationship (or a company for that matter) without challenge stops growing and becomes predictable, unprofitable, maybe even boring. Negotiation is paramount to the success of any two parties coming together for a mutual benefit.

In order to establish a truthful, intimate, and fulfilling relationship between yourself and someone you care about, you must negotiate a mutual advancement in the important

 "Love is cooperation rather than competition."

- Dr. Wayne Dyer

issues of your lives. Imagine your ultimate goals for a healthy and happy relationship leading to better physical and emotional health that then results in more job motivation with higher self-esteem and overall satisfaction.

NEURO-CISE: NEGOTIATING, DUO

As in business, you can apply the same principles to your romantic relationship:

- ♥ Write out honest, genuine needs you would like to see fulfilled by your partner and ask them to do the same.

♥ Discuss areas of concern that are least sensitive first.

♥ Clarify what new changes would look and feel like.

♥ Commit to changing the behaviors necessary to put the terms into effect.

You must address these issues from your point of view, not blaming the other person for what you do not get. Think about the times that your partner has done what you need and use those as examples to help them understand. "You know when I'm really tired after work, you tell me to sit back and relax while you rub my feet? I really appreciate your thoughtfulness!"

Get comfortable with the idea of scheduling a time to negotiate difficult matters by starting with less sensitive topics, such as who is going to take out the garbage or what time dinner will be during the week. Once you've figured out how to best maneuver those discussions, you can move to deeper issues like how often do you want to make love or where the kids should go to camp.

Make an agreement to listen carefully to your partner without being defensive or judgmental. When your partner has finished, repeat back what was said as closely as possible in your own words. You should ask open-ended questions such as, "What would you like from me?" "What did I do to make you feel that way?" or "Tell me more about that."

Don't start negotiating until the other partner is heard, and only then ask clarifying questions. For example, "When you said you'd like to make love four times a week, how would you feel about two of those times in the morning? You know how much I like to do it before going to the office!"

The conversation should continue until a resolution has been reached together that leaves both partners feeling satisfied. This would ideally involve equal compromise from both partners. At the end of the negotiation, schedule a specific time and place to follow up, in a few days or a week.

During the time until the follow up, a concerted effort needs to be made to keep to the agreement. The lines of communication need to remain open, regardless of what unexpected hurdles life may introduce. Just like a successful business, you need to invest your time and effort into a successful relationship, negotiate to achieve a win-win outcome, plan, collaborate, nurture your relationship and schedule quality time to share ideas in order to make it even better.

Fighting Fair

It's impossible to hope for a relationship that won't have disagreements. People are complicated. Life is challenging. Mistakes get made. Feelings get hurt. That's just the reality of what it means to be fully engaged in the grown up world.

> *"All men and women have an equal need for love. When these needs are not fulfilled it is easy to have our feelings hurt, for which we blame our partner."*
>
> *– Dr. John Gray*

The key to happiness isn't to avoid the fight but it's to learn how to lead with kindness and fight fair. However justified you may feel in blaming someone for something, it will simply lead to increased tension, resentment and defensiveness. Remember, fights are about feelings, so emotions will be raw. Be careful with your words and remember the rules of **I STILL LOVE YOU:**

Inhale. Exhale. Inhale. Exhale.

Stay away from "you always" and "you never."

Take time to listen.

Inhibit sarcasm.

Lead with "I feel" not "You are."

Let go of anger as fast as you can.

Leave the past in the past.

Offensive names are off limits.

Verify actions and intentions.

Encourage emotional understanding.

Yelling defeats the purpose.

Own up to mistakes.

Under the pain, is love.

Though it can feel awful to be in the middle of a disagreement, there are actually benefits to facing romantic conflict together. First and foremost, the fight isn't actually against each other as much as it is a fight for common ground. Both people are trying to pull their partner to their side. When it is done with respect, it should feel like tug of war, not dodge ball.

Healthy arguments can help create awareness about priorities and needs, which builds an intimate connection. Resolving issues together creates confidence in the relationship, leaving you both with the feeling that you are in this together and are willing to face whatever may come. Conflict resolution strengthens the romantic bond because each partner more intimately trusts that they can express their feelings and needs without the threat of abandonment.

A word of caution about make-up sex as I've known many passionate couples who create emotional drama just for the great sex that follows. In a healthy relationship, couples can share physical intimacy after a fight with the intention of resolution. Couples who say they love to fight to have make-up sex rarely create closure or resolution, so the negative emotions are always evident.

The Power Of Forgiveness

If communication is the key to a healthy relationship, then forgiveness is the door to be unlocked between a closed heart and an open one. Though it may feel like a gift to the person who has done us wrong, forgiveness is actually a gift you give to yourself. Lily Tomlin has a famous quote, "forgiveness means giving up all hope for a better past." Ultimately, forgiveness is the decision to let go of a grudge we're holding against someone who has caused us pain. This decision has nothing to do with condoning a negative action or taking steps to forgetting what has been done, it is simply making the choice to heal your own hurt.

If you question the validity of this, consider this experiment, as proposed by Dr. Elisha Goldstein, author of *The Now Effect*. Think of someone whom you are holding a grudge against right now, someone for whom forgiveness feels truly impossible. Picture that person, and pay attention to what emotions you feel. Anger? Resentment? Sadness? And what about your physical body? Is your jaw tight, fists clenched, stomach upset? You feel the emotional and physical effects of the negative memory, not the person who caused you pain. In the same way, releasing that pain through forgiveness heals your body and psyche but offers no relief to the other person. They don't even need to know that you forgive them because, again, it's not something you give away; it's something you give to yourself. You give yourself emotional freedom. In his book *Forgive for Good,* Dr. Fred Luskin states, "Forgiveness can be defined as the 'peace and understanding that come from blaming that which has hurt you less, taking the life experience less personally, and changing your grievance story.'"

"Forgiveness is the attribute of the strong."

–Mahatma Gandhi

In the short exercise we did a moment ago, the side effects of putting focus on the person we cannot forgive causes stress in the brain due to the resentment felt toward that particular person. Anxiety literally drains brain power, which causes the brain to go into protection mode, releasing cortisol. While very helpful in short-term protection, too much cortisol can actually shut down learning and cause depression. And long term surges have been linked to weakened immune systems, blood sugar imbalance and higher blood pressure.

A.J. Clark of the Department of Molecular and Cellular Biology at the University of Arizona described the biological and neurological components of forgiveness:

- ♥ Memories of the hurtful act arouse fear stemming from the amygdala (the memory center for fear and trauma).

- ♥ This fear drives a pattern of anger and fight-or-flight readiness (cortisol release).

- ♥ Under appropriate circumstances, the frontal cortex interrupts the pattern and quells the fear response in the amygdala.

- ♥ The resultant relaxation of muscular tension signals the cortex that forgiveness has occurred.

- ♥ The memory pathway from the rhinal cortex and hippocampus to the amygdala is inhibited.

- ♥ A tangible act confirms that the memories no longer stimulate the amygdala and the pattern of anger and stress does not occur.

As with most things, the path to forgiveness begins with the self. It may be easier to forgive those around us, but it is even more important to forgive our own mistakes. One simple exercise is to forgive yourself each week for the mistakes you made. Set aside a few minutes to review what went wrong, and how you might better have handled the situation.

A client of mine, Janet, has learned to stop wasting her time blaming others for what they have done to her. Instead, she opens up her weekly forgiveness ritual with something like this: "I forgive myself for going out on a blind date and expecting love at first sight" or

"I forgive myself for putting up with a man who belittled me." By forgiving herself in this manner, she remains focused on her needs rather than what is lacking in the other person. As Janet says, "When I release my resentments this way each week, it clears me up inside. I don't hear that rumble of anger underneath my breath anymore. And it helps me to stay focused on me and my expectations."

The grudges we hold against ourselves actually work as walls between the life we have and the life we want. If we don't feel worthy of our own forgiveness, it's hard to feel worthy of the greatness we desire, so we will either consciously or subconsciously hold it at bay. Only through forgiveness can we find the path to greatness. Recycled trash is still trash. You wouldn't dream of eating yesterday's garbage for dinner tonight, but that's similar to what you are doing if you keep recycling old hurts through your system. Forgiveness is daring to feel worthy of the love you seek, giving up what you may have accepted as love in the past, especially if it was wrong for you. Let's face it, as humans we are always going to make mistakes, but without mistakes there can be no forgiveness and without forgiveness, there can be no love!

NEURO-CISE: FORGIVENESS, DUO

Below are a few simple, but effective steps to help you clear the decks and move on. In order to rekindle passion, the first step is often forgiveness. Refusing to forgive can hurt you more than it hurts the other person. In my private practice when I help couples through the power of forgiveness, I ask the couple if any emotional, physical or sexual boundaries have been violated in their relationship. Then we discuss how it has affected the relationship and which ones are deal-breakers. Afterwards I counsel one person on how to ask for an apology from the other. For example, "I felt unappreciated and unloved when you were rude to me in public. It hurt my feelings and I need you to apologize to let me know how much you care about me." The guilty partner apologizes and takes responsibility and then they make a promise to never violate boundaries again.

1. Give up the grievance right away. Swallow your pride and don't waste your valuable energy dwelling on the wrongs done to you. When we forgive someone, we are healing ourselves within. We don't necessarily have to love, or even like someone in order to forgive him or her. Just do it and say it like you mean it.

2. Unload your backpack. Get rid of your hatreds and hurts before they congeal and petrify. Unload your emotional backpack; don't let it weigh you down and impede your quest for everlasting love. Talk to yourself in the mirror, talk to friends, a counselor, an empty chair, a stuffed animal, a movie star's photo, or even a pet. Just get the old emotions out in the open. Your anger can be constructive when properly channeled and constructively used to purge your pain. Hold the person you're angry with clearly in your mind. Then ask yourself, "What emotional shortcomings caused him or her to treat me badly?" This is what you want to have compassion for, and it is also the reason to forgive.

3. Expand forgiveness. Remember, forgiveness is not a one-time thing. You can forgive a person or situation again, as long as you do it quickly, rather than letting it fester.

4. Forgive yourself. Make it unconditional. Then let the situation go. Forgive yourself to find inner peace by letting go of the past and looking to the future creating new good memories to wipe away old bad ones. The Dalai Lama says, "Do not let the behavior of others destroy your inner peace."

5. To forgive somebody who isn't sorry is so hard that I recommend turning the pent up emotions of anger and pain into pity for the person's emotional cold heart. When you hate someone you give him or her control of your emotions. So, visualize opening up your heart and silently say to them, "I forgive you for everything you have done to hurt me." The forgiveness can be offered internally, with lasting healing

consequences for our own lives. The power of forgiveness has been shown to:

♥ Reduce hostility and stress.

♥ Relieve the toxic effects of unhealed emotional pain.

♥ Open one's ability to be more compassionate.

♥ Help one learn about themselves.

♥ Enhance one's ability to love unconditionally and get in touch with one's higher self.

♥ Help discover a sense of life purpose.

♥ Help to become "for-giving" to the community and the world as a whole.

♥ Strengthen one's ability to have satisfying, nurturing relationships.

♥ Increase one's sense of wholeness and bring forth a deep healing. This healing may include improvements in physical functioning of the body, healing of the emotions, healing of the mind and its belief-systems, and healing in relationships.

♥ Write a letter of forgiveness to each other for all the hurts you have both endured during your relationship. Read them out loud and say "thank you," then move on and let bygones be bygones.

Real-Life Revelation

Forgiveness played a huge part in the recovery of one of my clients. When Chad first came to me, he was an extremely angry man, trying to come to terms with his ex-partner's adultery. His pain was magnified by the fact that with the loss of the relationship, he also lost a connection with his ex's children. As a gay man, Chad wasn't sure fatherhood would ever be part of his story, though he had always longed for it, so he had tried to stay in the relationship with his ex in order to maintain his role as step-dad. Even though they had been going to couples counseling, the infidelity continued and Chad ultimately had to make the decision to protect his own heart and end the relationship, which also meant walking away from the kids he had grown to love as his own.

As Chad tried to work through his painful recovery, he learned that his ex had quickly moved on to a new relationship with the man with whom he had been cheating. In fact, they got married within four months of Chad ending the relationship.

To say the least, Chad wasn't exactly on board when I suggested that he had to find a way to forgive his ex-partner! His anger towards the loss of his old life was all-consuming and it seemed to fuel everything he did. He was enraged that his partner could so easily move on and he asked repeatedly how it was possible that someone like that could so quickly find happiness while Chad was left to suffer. He actually walked out of our session when I mentioned that he wasn't being made to suffer as much as he had made the choice to suffer.

I was pretty sure I wouldn't see Chad again, but he eventually called and apologized for storming out and asked to come in to see me. His next visit involved a confession that he hadn't previously shared: Chad's relationship with his ex had actually started while his ex was dating someone else. He had been the "other man" but chose to believe it wouldn't happen again and chose to ignore the subtle hints that it was happening because he liked being a dad and thought that would be enough to save the relationship. So while I had first told Chad that he had to learn to forgive his ex, I now realized that he had to forgive himself. He wasn't angry at the actions of his ex, he was mad at himself because he willingly entered a risky relationship. He selfishly wanted to be a dad without considering the pain he might cause the kids if the relationship didn't work out.

Once Chad saw the core of his resentment, he began the hard work of self-forgiveness. Forgiving his ex was much easier than he had expected because that wasn't where the true anger was pointed. The hardest exercise I had Chad do was to face himself in the mirror and say "I forgive you" repeatedly. He struggled with it for several weeks until one day he said it and looked at me with a startled expression and said, "I think I meant it that time."

While Chad had spent a lot of time trying to find the courage to face and forgive his ex, the ex became irrelevant once Chad forgave himself. He did write his ex a letter of forgiveness and then he invited me to the barbeque he had in his backyard with friends to burn it. The happy side note that I can share is that, as of this writing, Chad is dating again and he's in the beginning stages of adopting a child all on his own.

Installing the Good

Neuropsychologist Rick Hanson is the founder of the Wellspring Institute for Neuroscience and Contemplative Wisdom, as well as the author of several books, including The *Enlightened Brain* and *Hardwiring Happiness*. Much of Dr. Hanson's studies show how to work against what he defines as the brain's "negative bias."

As a protective device, the brain more readily recalls negative experiences in order to keep us from making similar mistakes. He goes so far as to say that the brain is like Velcro for negative experiences and like Teflon for

 "Focusing on the positive is like putting on contact lenses. It corrects our vision."

– Dr. Rick Hanson

positive experiences: the negative stick almost immediately while the positive need time to sink in. You will instantly remember that something burns you but an "average joy" such as the warmth of a crackling fire on a cold night must be held in the short-term memory for 10 to 20 seconds in order to settle into long-term storage.

There are three basis ways to engage the mind: live in the moment, release the negative and build up the positive. As Dr. Hanson describes it, "If the mind were a garden, we observe it, we pull weeds, and we plant flowers." When something negative happens, we first have to become aware of the undesirable feelings. We must notice the anger, hurt, sadness, or despair. With some time and work, we can move on to the phase of "pulling the weeds." It is here that we let go of the damage by removing it from the front and center of our consciousness. This is where Dr. Hanson believes most people stop. They forget to replace the removed negative with a positive. "As any gardener knows, if you pull weeds and don't plant flowers, the weeds will come back."

NEURO-CISE: GOOD MEMORY, SOLO

In order to embed happy experiences into our long-term memory ("plant the flowers", as it were), we must Notice, Focus and Install. To remember these steps, Dr. Hanson builds on the earlier analogy of fire:

1. **Light the fire**
   Notice a good experience that is happening or create a positive experience in the mind.

2. **Add logs to the fire**
   Stay with the experience or thought. Give it to yourself. Let your focus on it last 10-20 seconds and do this repeatedly throughout the day.

3. **Be warmed by the fire**
   Absorb the positive experience by acknowledging that it is going into you.

Yours and Mine, Entwined

Overcoming obstacles together is how you know the love is real. It's easy to love someone when life is going well, but when you survive the storms of change and challenge together, that's when you know you've found someone special and you can rekindle passion that may have faded. Sometimes you see the storm clouds coming and you have time to stock the shelves and board up the windows before the wind starts to howl. Other times you're struck by an earthquake that splits open the earth that you thought was so solid. Regardless of what comes along, there's comfort in knowing there's someone along for the ride with you. The skies might sometimes get gloomy but there's shelter in the heart of a true partner.

When the tests of life come along, it's important to know how to face them. Join me in the next chapter as we examine some of these tests and work toward Finding The Light In The Dark.

CHAPTER EIGHT
Finding the Light in the Dark

The cold, hard truth is that sometimes love hurts. To be fully invested in the acts of love in a romantic relationship means that you need to be open to the inevitable dark energies. Like the balance of light and dark, hot and cold, or positive and negative, Yin and Yang are the two essential principles of love. As I mentioned in the Tantra section, the Yin force is commonly associated with femininity, focusing on slow sensuality, while the Yang force is often dominant in masculinity, focusing more on the climax rather than the journey. But to experience the full enjoyment of love, the male and female forces must be balanced (regardless of actual gender) with a combination of both Yin and Yang energy.

To say that men are all one way and women are another is too simplistic. We can generalize

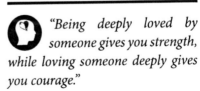 *"Being deeply loved by someone gives you strength, while loving someone deeply gives you courage."*

– Lao Tzu

by saying that many women display predominantly feminine characteristics, such as being sensual, passive, nurturing, loving, vulnerable, sensitive, compassionate, and receptive, while men display masculine qualities such as being sexual, active, controlling, strong, confident, assertive and protective. Yet, in some successful relationships, the woman is the masculine force and the man more feminine. Same sex relationships work the same way. The important thing is to achieve balance, which creates harmony.

Harmony is challenged by many factors: disappointment, anger, fear, stress, guilt, financial problems, power struggles, addiction, infidelity, and miscommunication are all common sources of discord. Any of these issues can unravel a relationship, but if you put forth enough effort to find the root cause of conflict and resolve it, your relationship will become stronger. And if you discover that a break up is the best option, at least you can say you tried your best and didn't just give up.

Crisis Can Deepen Love

Many of my clients come to see me when their relationship is in crisis. After all, why seek counseling when things are going smoothly? I always tell them that trauma can deepen their relationship bond, as it did for me in my personal life.

My husband and I suffered a horrific, dramatic event that ultimately brought us closer together. He was savagely attacked in our garage and left for dead with a knife wound across his neck from ear to ear and slashed across the chest from shoulder to rib cage barely missing his heart, but Peter managed to stumble into our house before he collapsed. I left the back door open for him and had no idea that he had saved my life by not letting the assailants cord-cuff his wrists because he knew that they would torture and kill us if they got into our home. I was terrified seeing him bleeding to death, hit the alarm button of our security system, and called 911. Then I quickly applied a towel to his neck as a tourniquet to try to staunch the bleeding. We later realized that my efforts and quick thinking saved his life.

Adding to my profound trauma, the police treated me as a suspect, hypothesizing that I had some connection to the assailants, which was devastating.

About a week later, detectives found an abandoned rental van that had been partially burned with my husband's credit cards and driver's license inside, which led them to the man behind the attack, a psychopathic former client of my husband, who is a criminal defense attorney. Peter had represented the man for burglary and knew he was capable of violence, but never told me that he had threatened him in court and at his office. I was angry when I found out about that last detail, but certainly couldn't lash out at my husband who was still recovering in the hospital. So I wrote Peter a letter describing my resentments in detail and ended it with my unconditional love and forgiveness. When I read it to him, he thanked me.

One of the most important things to do in the process of drawing closer together is learning to forgive. Visualize your love healing your partner's wounds, and your partner's love energy healing you. Writing a letter is one example of "taking out the emotional trash" in our lives, but of course there are many ways to release pent-up pain and negativity on the way to forgiveness.

> "I really do think that any deep crisis is an opportunity to make your life extraordinary in some way."
>
> – Martha Beck

Don't Be Afraid Of Fear

It has been said that humans ultimately only have two emotions, love and fear, and that every other emotion is merely a sub-category of either of these. For instance, on the love side you will find peace, happiness, forgiveness and joy, while the fear side is home to hate, depression, guilt, anxiety, and anger. If this is true, learning to understand and manage fear gives us the tools to change any negative emotion.

That's not to say that all fear is bad. If you come home from work to find a grizzly bear standing in your living room, it's good to have the internal warning signals to take appropriate actions to keep safe! But other fears are counterproductive to reaching personal, professional and romantic goals, such as fear of intimacy, speaking in front of crowds, or being perceived as foolish.

> *"There are two basic motivating forces: fear and love. When we are afraid, we pull back from life. When we are in love, we open to all that life has to offer with passion, excitement, and acceptance."*
>
> *– John Lennon*

There are four areas of the brain that help process the emotions associated with fear:

1. The hippocampus, sensory cortex, and amygdala examine each new situation and decipher if fear is a proper response.

2. The thalamus works as a control center, directing these signals to other parts of the brain.

3. The fight-or-flight response is activated in the hypothalamus, which notifies the adrenal glands to release stress hormones.

4. The frontal and temporal lobes release dopamine, which can lead to feelings of dread and panicked, illogical behavior.

Once the brain triggers an emotional response to fear, it becomes a full-body experience. In preparation for an increase in physical demands, the heart begins beating faster in order to pump more blood to the large muscles that may be called into action. Since some of the largest muscles are in the legs, and our subconscious mind is preparing for the possibility of a need to run, the muscle tension can cause our legs to shake. We also sweat in preparation for cooling off a body under duress.

The phenomenon of goose bumps, scientifically referred to as piloerection, causes the hairs on arms and legs to stand up. Though there is little understanding why this happens, it's quite possibly a holdover from our hairier ancestors for whom this response could cause them to puff up and look bigger to ward off a threat, much like a cat does.

NEURO-CISE: FEAR, SOLO

The more fully engaged we are in life, the more fears we are likely to have, because not only do we feel fear when we are threatened, we also feel it when we put ourselves at risk. And what is life without risk? To make a commitment to avoid fear would mean to turn your back on love, adventure, social change, and personal growth. So the answer isn't to remove fear as much as learn how to manage it. Treated with respect, fear can be transformed into wings that let you **SOAR**.

Simplify

Fear can quickly turn a breeze into a hurricane. Shake the fear down to its most basic root so it can be seen clearly for what it is. "I'm scared of going on a blind date" is a large-scale issue that can feel overwhelming and create a shutdown to the possibility. If you ask yourself "Why?" repeatedly and answer honestly, it's quite possible that you will find a small, manageable dread that can be addressed, and alleviate what feels like an epic fear.

Observe

Once you find the core issue that is causing you to panic, look for the warning that it is trying to give you. Most fears are based in past experiences that caused pain or discomfort at the time. The brain is trying to protect you from repeating a painful situation. Sometimes these memories are not even from your own experience, just a "horror story" you have seen or heard about. Remind yourself that every experience is a new opportunity and no two outcomes will ever be the same. Your best friend's awful blind date is not a guarantee that yours will be bad as well.

Accept

The Outward Bound Program has this great motto: "The goal is not to rid our stomachs of butterflies, but to get them to fly in formation!" We must acknowledge that feeling fear is a part of life, but that doesn't mean we must live fearfully. When we decipher what base issue is causing the internal strife, we can accept it. "I accept that I'm nervous about this blind date, but I'm more nervous to miss an opportunity to find love, so I'm going to go."

Release

All fears are based in apprehension about a possible future outcome, even when that future is as close as a few minutes from now. When you are overcome with fear, you are no longer in the moment; your brain is trying to protect you from an imagined future. If you take the time to see the fear clearly for what it is, you take the control away from the fear and allow for mindful decisions. So, "My blind date is late. She or he already hates me," becomes "My blind date is late. Excellent. I have a few extra minutes to review today's news so we'll have more to talk about."

Turning Guilt into Gilt

Guilt is always complicated, rarely welcome and never kind. Are you conscious of the guilt in your own life? I have yet to meet anyone who lives completely guilt-free, regardless of how carefree they

 "Guilt is anger directed at ourselves - at what we did or did not do."

– Peter McWilliams

may appear. Turning guilt into gilt is indeed a golden challenge, whether it's a feeling of being remiss in our duty to another person or an unnecessary load of "excess-baggage guilt." But one thing's for sure, the more guilt you can get rid of, the more you will enjoy life.

The brain processes guilt in the prefrontal cortex where messages of losses and gains are assessed as part of the reward center. When the messages from an action are tallied, and the brain makes the final call that the losses outnumber the gains, a sense of guilt is created, a feeling of unease about decisions made or actions taken. When this activity is repeated excessively, the uneasy feelings become burdensome, especially in people who are insecure.

There is a very strong correlation in the brain between guilt and depression. One negative action or mistake can spawn numerous unnecessary guilt attacks within ourselves. As Dr. Roland Zahn, a clinical neuroscientist at The University of Manchester's School of Psychological Sciences, states, "The most distinctive feature of depressive disorders is an exaggerated negative attitude to oneself, which is typically accompanied by feelings of guilt."

There are also medical findings indicating that guilt is anger directed internally. A study done by the National Institutes of Neurological Disorders that was subsequently published in the journal *Cerebral Cortex*, examined the way the brain responded to questions of social behavior. When faced with behaviors they felt were morally wrong, the subjects displayed anger toward actions performed by others, but guilt when expressing feelings about their own questionable behavior.

One of my clients was an overly cautious woman named Gretchen whose life had been taken over by guilt. Several years before she had come to see me, Gretchen was faced with a choice between going home for Christmas or traveling with her girlfriend to Italy for the holidays. Though her mother begged her to come home, Gretchen made the choice to take the vacation instead. Tragically, her grandmother passed away in the week after Christmas and Gretchen had to cut her vacation short in order to attend the funeral. Her mother didn't help the situation by reprimanding Gretchen for being so selfish as to take the Italian trip instead of coming home, knowing how important Christmas was to her grandmother and reminding her repeatedly that she missed the opportunity to say good-bye. Gretchen had become so tormented by guilt that she was willing to punish herself by relocating back to her hometown in order to be close to her mother.

In order to turn guilt into gold, we must practice acceptance and forgiveness of ourselves, and offer it to the people around us. We cannot control what we are given. We can only control how we choose to respond and, in many cases, guilt is a form of unexpressed grief. This was the case for Gretchen. More than the hurtful things her mother would say, Gretchen was truly devastated that she didn't have an opportunity to tell her grandmother good-bye, a woman who had been a huge, positive influence in her life.

While visiting her mother and making further plans to move back to her hometown, I asked Gretchen to take an afternoon to visit her grandmother's grave and say the things she would have said if she were still alive. This simple act of expressing her remorse as well as her gratitude gave Gretchen a tremendous sense of relief. Returning from the cemetery, she gave her mother a big hug and then sat her down to express how she was feeling and that she was tired of feeling guilty. Her mother apologized profusely, having no real understanding of how her own grief was being displayed passive-aggressively. Needless to say, Gretchen's mother told her daughter there was no need for her to uproot her life to move back home.

Overcoming unnecessary feelings of guilt begins with the difficult task of forgiveness. It is not possible to undo what has been done, it is only possible to move forward mindfully with a commitment to learn and respect the life lessons we are given.

Anger Is A Boomerang
Even more damaging than guilt, anger has the potential to manifest itself in truly violent ways such as mental, physical and sexual abuse. We're all familiar with how anger feels. It's an incredibly powerful emotion. When managed in a healthy way, it can be a fantastic motivator as it signals that something is wrong and inspires us to make changes, both in the short-term (leaving a stressful situation) or the long-term (finding a better job). However, when anger goes unchecked, it can have devastating consequences.

One of the nation's leading experts on anger, Dr. Howard Kassinove defines anger as "a negative feeling state that is typically associated with hostile thoughts, physiological arousal and maladaptive behaviors. It usually develops in response

"Holding on to anger is like grasping a hot coal with the intent of throwing it at someone else; you are the one who gets burned."

- Buddha

to the unwanted actions of another person who is perceived to be disrespectful, demeaning, threatening or neglectful." The most prominent response to anger is retaliation, partly because the area of the brain responsible for logic literally shuts down during feelings of anger.

Signals from the outside world are sent to the amygdala where it is decided if the information should be processed by the limbic (emotional) or cortex (logic) portion of the brain. If these messages fire off enough emotional sparks, the amygdala will override the cortex's message of judgment and evaluation and release a flood of the stress hormones adrenaline and cortisol that cause emotional and physical alarm. This energy eruption sets off a fight or flight response that causes the muscles to tense up in preparation for action, the heart rate to increase and blood pressure to elevate as breathing becomes faster. This increase in oxygen to the brain makes it harder to think clearly and, because logic and the contemplation of consequences are being stifled, words and actions may be used that will later be regretted when the thinking part of the brain is again allowed to process more fully. It can take between 20 and 60 minutes for the body and brain to return to a balanced state.

Aggression is often times the "bully brother" of anger that aims to harm. It represents the desire to control and dominate a person or situation and can be expressed with violent words and actions. Punching, shoving, hitting, screaming, belittling, and mocking are all manifestations of anger.

Not only is anger something we inflict on others, but it also has physical repercussions in our own bodies. Rage issues are linked to asthma, heart disease, and chronic pain. Dr. Kassinove further explains the long term effects of excessive anger: "These physiological reactions can lead to increases in cardiovascular responding, in respiration and perspiration, in blood flow to active muscles and in strength. As the anger persists, it will affect many of the body's systems, such as the cardiovascular, immune, digestive and central nervous systems. This will lead to increased risks of hypertension and stroke, heart disease, gastric ulcers, and bowel diseases, as well as slower wound healing."

NEURO-CISE: TAME YOUR TEMPER, SOLO

Learning to control and diffuse your anger can be extremely challenging, but it's a necessary step in maintaining personal and interpersonal health. The Mayo Clinic offers these ideas as a way to keep anger in check:

1. **Take a timeout**
   No, timeouts aren't just for kids. Taking a moment to breathe by counting to 10 allows the brain to relax enough to generate a more mindful response to aggravations.

2. **Once you're calm, express your anger**
   Do not try to suppress or deny angry feelings. Express them in a clear but nonjudgmental way using respectful language.

3. **Get some exercise**
   Physical activity creates an outlet for emotions that may be dangerous to express in a more explosive way. Brain chemicals are stimulated that create feelings of happiness and relaxation, allowing for a gentler response.

4. **Think before you speak**
   Though it's tempting to give an immediate response when confronted with frustration, consider this: it's easier to say the

right thing first than to ask for forgiveness later, after the heat of the moment led to a regretful response. It's better to prevent damage, than try to change it after the fact.

5. **Identify possible solutions**
   If a situation seems to repeatedly lead to feelings of anger, analyze the situation to see if there are ways to correct it, possibly with adjustments, acceptance or compromise.

6. **Stick with 'I' statements**
   Blame will only increase tension, so it's important to be respectful and specific while discussing a tense situation with "I" statements. "I'm upset that you were late getting home from work" will be met with a more open mind than "You are never on time."

7. **Don't hold a grudge**
   Holding onto anger plants a seed of bitterness that can forever taint how you view a person or situation. Only through genuine forgiveness can you truly unclench the fist of resentment.

8. **Use humor to release tension**
   You can let the air out of a tense situation by utilizing humor. You must, however, be careful to avoid sarcasm or passive aggressive remarks that can only make things worse.

9. **Practice relaxation skills**
   Finding the tools that help you relax can go a long way to saving a tense situation. Breathing exercises, visualization, yoga poses, or calming mantras such as "I am not my anger" can all come to the rescue when things get difficult.

10. **Know when to seek help**
    If you find that anger is becoming an increasing challenge to manage, it's extremely important to seek assistance before serious damage is done. With the aid of professional help, you

can thoroughly examine the root of your triggers, learn to react responsibly and explore any underlying issues that may be unresolved.

Dealing With Depression

There are few emotional states more debilitating than depression. It's a truly devastating illness that can destroy relationships and potentially lead to suicidal thoughts and actions. The good news is that depression is

> "A woman should not persist in trying to draw a man's feelings out when he is angry or upset."
>
> – Dr. John Gray

treatable. The challenging news is that the work must begin with the inflicted person recognizing their own illness and making a conscious decision to go to war against it, which can be difficult when self-worth and energy are low.

An over-production of cortisol has been found in severely depressed patients, leading some psychiatrists to view acute depression as a kind of long-term stress on the body. It is not believed that cortisol is the cause of this illness as much as it is a consequence of extended psychological distress.

One aspect of life that is usually undermined by depression is sexual intimacy. For many people, a depressed state of mind causes them to lose interest in sex while others who find that sex is the only thing that makes them feel better.

Side effects of depression can include excessive exhaustion or insomnia, changes in eating habits, lack of concentration, and a growing apathy toward life in general. The condition is surprisingly common, with as many as one in five people facing some form of a depressive order at some time in their lives. Treatment ranges from psychotherapeutic to chemical. Most antidepressants utilize selective serotonin reuptake inhibitors (SSRIs), as it is believed that a serotonin imbalance is at the chemical core of chronic depression. Not only are levels low, but some serotonin is being reabsorbed too soon by the body, resulting in impaired brain cell communication. The effects of SSRIs can be felt rapidly, usually within a couple weeks, though the benefits are greatly increased with additional life work such as psychotherapy, diet, exercise and positive changes to circumstances and surroundings.

Though one of the most debilitating aspects of depression can be exhaustion, the best treatment is a course of action. The key is to set goals that are easy to accomplish so you don't devastate yourself with disappointment when large goals prove to be overwhelming. "I'm going to wash the dishes everyday" is much more obtainable than "I'm going to repaint my bedroom this weekend." Even a most basic routine can help start you back on track. Endorphins have also proven to have long-term benefits for the fight against depression, so exercise is a great defense. Again, keep the objectives simple. Walk around the block twice a week before you decide to train for a triathlon.

> "You largely constructed your depression. It wasn't given to you. Therefore, you can deconstruct it."
>
> – Dr. Albert Ellis

Dopamine is the brain's antidepressant as it's associated with pleasure, gratification and education. One way to alter dopamine levels is to do something new. Learning inspires chemical changes in the brain, so go to a museum, read a book, volunteer to work with children or an animal rescue, take a class and learn a new hobby. It may sound odd, but when you're depressed you have to relearn how to have fun. Make a list of the things you used to enjoy and start doing some of them again, even if it feels like a chore. Eventually the smiles will come easier and the clouds will dissipate.

NEURO-CISE: ANTI-DEPRESSION, SOLO

Here are ten steps to help you battle depression:

1. Identify when and what triggers your depression and let your partner, family or friends know so that they are prepared before it happens.

2. Make a list of all the things that you are most grateful for and keep it close by so that you can look at it as a daily ritual.

3. Get out of your home or office, even if it's just for a short walk, preferably with your partner or a friend. Go to support groups, the mall, out to eat, the movies or any place where you can be socially active.

4. Take care of yourself physically. Get up, bathe each day and eat nutritious foods. Do not abuse your body by under eating or over eating.

5. Make your heart sing by doing something that makes you laugh or smile. Watch a funny TV show or movie, play with a dog or cat, watch kids play at a playground, go to the zoo, or listen to good music.

6. Do not neglect intimacy, even if you don't feel like having sex. If you are in a relationship, let your partner know how much you appreciate him or her. Hold, kiss and caress each other because your brain will release pleasure endorphins that will rapidly elevate your mood. If you're unattached romantically, pleasuring yourself will give you the same flood of feel-good endorphins.

7. Believe that your depression will be replaced with happiness and make a daily habit of visualizing yourself enjoying life again.

8. Don't blame others for the way you feel.

9. When you are having a bad day, let people know not to worry because things will get better.

10. Don't give up hope and feel sorry for yourself. Be strong and replace negative thoughts with positive ones.

NEURO-CISE: ANTI-DEPRESSION, DUO

As a partner of someone battling depression, there are many steps you can take to help win the war:

1. Encourage your partner to get all the professional help available.

2. Offer supportive words, but do not show pity.

3. Emphasize your partner's good qualities, especially when he or she is feeling down.

4. Help your partner stay socially and physically active by taking them out in public and walking or exercising together.

5. Listen and be as patient as if your partner was recovering from surgery.

6. Don't despair or blame yourself for your partner's depression.

7. Believe that your partner's depression will be replaced with happiness and visualize the two of you enjoying life again.

8. Maintain intimacy with lots of hugging.

9. Take time to value and reward yourself for being such a loving and caring person.

10. Let your partner know how much you love them and that you will always be there for them.

Mommy News For Baby Blues

One of depression's evil step-sisters affects 80% of new mothers within the first 10 days of giving birth. Dubbed the "baby blues," it brings with it mild depression interspersed with happy feelings and a variety of symptoms including fatigue, sadness, crying spells, anxiety, confusion, oversensitivity, loneliness, and sleep disorders. Given the extraordinary physical and chemical changes that go through the female body before, during and after childbirth—combined with the arrival of a screaming, pooping, peeing, hyper-dependent new little human—it's not exactly surprising that these things happen, and they generally subside within two weeks.

When these "blues" persist and/or intensify, they cross the line into clinical Postpartum Depression (PPD). As many as 20% of new mothers will experience PPD. Onset can occur anytime during the first year after delivery and it may last from three to 14 months, or even longer. Though many symptoms are similar to major depressive disorder, many are unique to PPD, including extreme anger, guilt, fear, obsessive thoughts of inadequacy as a parent, disconnection from the baby, and loss of control of one's life.

In trying to understand this disease, a study at the University of Pittsburg points to findings that metabolism in the amygdala was considerably different in women with PPD than those without it, though it is unclear if these differences are the cause or the effect of postpartum depression.

As part of the limbic system and associated with functions related to memory, nervousness and fear, among other emotions, any amygdala dysfunctions would be associated with anxiety disorders, borderline personality disorder, and posttraumatic stress disorder. As part of the system that releases stress hormones, this area of the brain also has an effect on the sympathetic nervous system and jumpstarts the fight or flight response.

The same University of Pittsburgh study also shows that mothers afflicted with PPD symptoms had less amygdala reaction in the areas associated with empathy and protective response when presented with images of sad or upset people and children, but an increase in the area associated with hostility. This helps us understand why women with PPD struggle so much to connect with their babies.

While suffering postpartum depression can be devastating, it is equally confusing and difficult for the new mother's partner to make sense of the grief in what should be a joyous occasion. Dr. Karen Kleiman, founder of The Postpartum

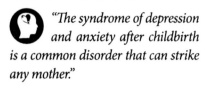

"The syndrome of depression and anxiety after childbirth is a common disorder that can strike any mother."

– Dr. Karen Kleiman

Stress Center, and author of several books on the subject, offers a lot of practical information on dealing with PPD as both the new mother and the partner try to understand what's going on. She says the most important things are to take this very seriously and to learn as much as you can about the subject while getting professional help. Also, keep these tips in mind:

- ♥ Be aware that her emotional vulnerability may get in the way of good communication.

- ♥ Set limitations with friends and family.

- ♥ Help around the house.

- ♥ Accompany her to doctor's appointments.

- ♥ Try to postpone any important decision until after she is feeling better.

- ♥ Intervene so she can get uninterrupted sleep.

Dr. Kleiman says that ultimately the most important thing that you can do to help is to simply be there for your suffering partner. "Sit with her. No TV, no kids, no dog, no bills, no newspaper. Just you and her. Let her know you're there. This isn't easy to do, especially with someone who seems so sad or so distant. Five minutes a day is a good place to start."

PPD is not only a risk for the female who gave birth but also her partner. It is estimated that 10% of the partners of new mothers are afflicted with postpartum symptoms of their own. With or without postpartum issues, a newborn (and the demands of children in general) can take a toll on a person's sex drive, which can result in an imbalance in desire.

Understanding Infidelity

Looking to better understand why cheating happens, I conducted a survey through my own Loveology University with the help of Dr. Leanna Wolfe, an anthropologist and researcher. With over 1,000 respondents from both sides of the discussion, both sexes and a full spectrum of ages, we gained some interesting insight into adultery.

Our results showed that 61% had been cheated on, 59% had cheated on a partner and 57% had been secret partners, so as you can see, many of our respondents had been part

"Infidelity raises profound questions about intimacy."

– Junot Diaz

of all three corners of this triangle. We were able to draw gender conclusions with some dramatic differences between how men and women define cheating. Men are more likely to define cheating as genital contact, whereas women consider emotional connections, such as having dinner, to be cheating as well.

- ♥ Males define cheating when there is genital contact.

- ♥ Males cheat for excitement.

- ♥ Males cheat to live out their sexual fantasies.

- ♥ Males believe they can get away with cheating.

- ♥ Females consider emotional connection to be cheating.

- ♥ Females cheat for attention.

- ♥ Female secret partners find less satisfaction.

- ♥ Females are more likely to consider cheating to be wrong.

Beyond gender, age was also a big factor in determining reasons for cheating. In both sexes that participated in my survey, those under 35 were most likely to cheat for attention. Those over 35 were most likely to cheat in pursuit of sexual variety, wanting something their partner at home was not giving them. What this means is that there are ways to help ensure that the bonds of fidelity are not broken.

My personal opinion may not be popular, but I do not believe that monogamy is a natural human phenomenon. Instead, it is a choice that we make as part of a commitment to another person in a romantic relationship. Infidelity does not need to be the end of the world. As heartbreaking as it can be, I believe it is a wound that can be healed, and relationships that endure it can survive.

NEURO-CISE: 10 WAYS TO REDUCE THE RISK OF INFIDELITY

1. Kiss each other passionately daily.

2. Remain curious about each other's lives.

3. Don't keep secrets from each other.

4. Nip problems in the bud when they occur.

5. Avoid tempting situations with someone you find attractive.

6. Communicate about your wants, needs, desires and fantasies.

7. Always show appreciation for your partner.

8. Don't neglect your partner, especially on special occasions.

9. Keep the flames of passion burning by creating romantic memories.

10. Respect your partner by being polite in any situation.

An important step in a romantic relationship is to make sure you are aware of your partner's definition of cheating. For instance, is it possible for a lunch or dinner to be considered cheating? What about dirty dancing at a club? A kiss on the cheek? A closed mouth kiss on the lips? What about emotional intimacy and or cybersex? Some survey respondents considered all of these things cheating. BDSM, phone sex and happy ending massage are all services that you can pay for. So are G-spot and prostate massage when you visit a sex surrogate. Is that cheating? And finally, sexual intercourse, oral sex and anal sex are considered cheating virtually by everyone, but there are some people willing to make exceptions in certain circumstances.

> *"There exists no culture in which adultery is unknown, no cultural device or code that extinguishes philandering."*
>
> – Dr. Helen Fisher

To some (especially women), infidelity is defined as "emotional cheating," making it easier to accept a partner's sexual indiscretion more so than what is perceived as a romantic connection, even if sex isn't part of the latter equation.

There are many solutions to help you recover from a cheating partner that will enable you to have the kind of healthy relationship that you deserve. One such exercise is to write a Profit & Loss Relationship Statement. On the Profit Side, list all of your partner's positive qualities and the advantages of staying together. On the Loss Side, list all of your partner's negative qualities and the reasons why splitting up would be better.

Regardless of the outcome of this exercise, it's important that you don't blame or punish yourself by drinking, binge eating or starving, medicating or hurting yourself. This won't change the circumstances and could possibly make matters worse. It's equally necessary that you don't rush to tell your family and friends about the cheating until you have all the facts. They may hold lasting grudges that cannot be repaired and this can cause much unneeded strife, especially if you choose to stay together and work to get your relationship back on track.

The cheating brain is hungry for dopamine that spikes when a new stimulus excites their radar. So what keeps a brain from cheating? The 'cuddle hormone' oxytocin helps, as the more we experience, the more we bond to that person and the more likely we are to stay monogamous.

Addicted To Love

"Addicted to Love" was a hit song for Robert Palmer in 1985 and remains a perennial pop favorite today, but the reality of love addiction isn't so much fun.

Being in love feels fantastic but not when it crosses into obsessive thinking, manipulation, crippling fear, and panic attacks. If self-worth and happiness all hinge on a romantic relationship, it places a stranglehold on a healthy life. This overwhelming need, this starvation for love, thrives on a dangerous blend of high expectations and low self-esteem. The 'love addict' begs for a love that he or she feels unworthy of, creating a no-win situation.

In her book, *Love Addict: Sex, Romance, and Other Dangerous Drugs,* Ethlie Ann Vare offers incredible insight into the rarely discussed affliction of love addiction. By using alcoholism as a comparison, she found that many of the psychological and behavioral issues were the same, which indicates that, like the difference between a heavy drinker and an alcoholic, there is a difference between someone who loves love and a love addict. There really isn't a strict test to decipher if you're a love addict, but Ethlie offers a series of statements to consider that may indicate a problem. Here are 10 of them:

1. I often feel an instant connection to someone I've just met.

2. I consistently choose partners who are emotionally, geographically, or logistically unavailable.

3. I have passed over family, social or career opportunities in favor of romantic and sexual ones.

4. I use sex to hook a prospective romantic partner.

5. I have considered, threatened or attempted suicide over a relationship.

6. I feel worthless when I am not in a relationship and jump into the next one as quickly as possible.

7. When I'm attracted to someone, I often ignore warning signs that this person isn't good for me.

8. I am possessive and jealous when I'm in love.

9. I like to be the pursuer in the game of love, even chasing after people who have rejected me.

10. I have been dependent on drugs, alcohol, gambling, spending or food in the past, but most people think I have my life together.

Again, this is not a scientific test and it's actually possible to answer "yes" to all of them and not be addicted to love. However, your gut reaction to the questions and the intensity with which you can answer "yes" is a good indication of whether or not you should take a closer

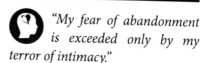

"My fear of abandonment is exceeded only by my terror of intimacy."

- Ethlie Ann Vare

look. The concept of love addiction is incredibly complicated, largely because it is so hard to understand. As Ethlie puts it, "Sex and love aren't the problem. They are someone's solution to a problem we don't understand."

As described by doctors Harvey Milkman and Stanley Sunderwirth in their book, *Craving for Ecstasy: The Consciousness and Chemistry of Escape,* the brain's reward system has three divisions:

1. **Arousal:** gambling, cocaine, extreme sports, sex
2. **Satiation:** overeating, alcohol, heroin, relationship attachment
3. **Fantasy:** LSD, marijuana, religion, and romance

Romantic relationship elements are the only ones that cross all three divisions, making love addiction quite intense. What helps define behavior as an addiction is the obsessive element. A desire for love is replaced with an obsessive need for love that can lead to stalking tendencies, excessive relationship "hoping," and mistaking every "hello" as an invitation for romance.

The brain chemicals most associated with love addiction are dopamine, serotonin, vasopressin, oxytocin, and phenyl- ethylamine (PEA), with others like testosterone and adrenaline coming into the mix as well. While all of these elements play a big part in a healthy romantic relationship, it is the miscommunication between these elements within the addict's brain that causes problems. In *Healing the Addicted Brain,* Dr. Harold Urschel uses the analogy of a phone call to describe how this miscommunication happens:

If one cell is trying to speak to another cell but doesn't have enough of the necessary neurotransmitters, it can only whisper its message or even become mute. If it has too much of certain neurotransmitters, it may send an incorrect message. Conversely, if a cell is trying to listen to another cell but doesn't have the proper assistance, it will only hear the message faintly, if at all. Or, if the cell has too many of a certain receptor, it will ignore the messages of others. It's not an imbalance that happens as much as the addict brain isn't using what it has properly. The trigger, whether it is cocaine or a new relationship, gives a short-term boost to these transmitters, causing a chain reaction through the brain's reward center, which in turn creates a hunger for these euphoric feelings.

Love addicts can feel a gaping hole in the center of their lives when they are not in a relationship. It is in his or her nature to quickly, desperately find the next partner, simply to have someone, anyone, to give their life meaning. It is easy to focus on the potential of something instead of the reality of it. You must look at your situation as an outsider and examine the facts as they are today. Is this relationship healthy? Are my needs being met? Have I accidentally placed my partner on a pedestal? Are we equals or am I the only one willing to compromise?

Sadly, making the choice to stop loving in an unhealthy way may result in the need to end a damaging relationship. A partner, who has been treated like royalty, with no need for compromise or equality, may not know how to give you the healthy relationship you need. Even the end of a bad relationship needs a grieving process. It helps cleanse the psyche so the same negative patterns don't get repeated. Give yourself time to fully feel the loss and try to find the positive things that you can take away from the experience.

Addicted To Sex

Enjoying sex certainly isn't a cause for concern, nor is a desire to have sex often. However, there is a line that can be crossed when desire becomes an obsession and that's when things become troublesome and dangerous.

Sex addiction afflicts someone that has a compulsive sexual disorder with no (or little) self-control. It is believed that as many as 30 million people in the United States suffer from some level of sexual addiction. Consider the following questions that are used to define someone's level of addiction:

1. Do you think about sex so often that it interferes with your concentration?

2. Are you obsessed with a specific person or sexual act even though it brings you cravings and discomfort?

3. Are you finding your sexual pursuits affect your ability to manage your life?

4. Do you HAVE to flirt?

5. Do you feel you are entitled to sex?

6. Would life have no meaning without sex?

7. Do you think that sex is the only thing that really gives you value?

8. Do you use sex as an escape from other problems or stress?

9. Do you keep a list of the partners you have been with?

10. Do you need the "high" that the dangerous sex and the risk of being caught can promise?

If your answer to all these questions is "yes", then you possibly suffer from sexual compulsion. Sexual addiction is a relatively new addition to psychosexual disorders. People were simply defined as being hyper-sexual, players, promiscuous, and not wired for monogamy. It was as recent as 1983 that sexual addiction first came to the front and center of the news as a legitimate medical concern upon the publication of *Out of the Shadows: Understanding Sexual Addiction* by Dr. Patrick Carnes. These hyper-sexual behaviors are oftentimes connected to other addictive or obsessive personality traits, psychological disorders, self-esteem issues, self-destructive behavior, hereditary addiction issues, and lowered sexual inhibitions.

A sexual addict's mind is sparked the same way as most addictions occur. The brain tells the sex addict that having illicit sex is good the same way it tells over-eaters that over eating is good. The addicted brain fools the body by producing intense biochemical rewards (levels of PEA phenylethylamine) that boost euphoria for self-destructive behavior. There are three-stage progressions in becoming addicted:

> "*Sexual addicts are willing to sacrifice what they cherish most in order to preserve and continue their unhealthy behavior.*"
>
> – Dr. Patrick Carnes

1. In the first stage, the person actually believes that his or her addiction is healthy, normal, and pleasurable.

2. In the second stage, the person has conflicting thoughts about whether or not the addiction is healthy, normal, and pleasurable.

3. In the third stage, the person realizes that they are addicted and feels unhealthy, abnormal, and more pain than pleasure, yet he or she maintains and feeds the addiction.

The key is to discover the thought processes that are at the base of the addictive behavior and working to replace them with healthy behavior or eradicate them. Trauma, grief, previous abuse, anxiety and depression have all been linked to sexual addiction. In these cases, the act of intercourse is not treated as something sexual, it becomes medicinal. The endorphins, serotonin and testosterone of sexual activity and release create the bandage that briefly soothes the deeper, untreated pain.

The four most common methods for treating sexual addiction are the same as treatments for any other addictions:

1. The Twelve Step Programs

2. Psychotherapy

3. Sex Addiction Treatment Facilities

4. Spiritual Intervention

Like food addictions, sexual addiction can be challenging to treat because sex is an important part of life. It's our second basic instinct after survival, and unlike learning to function without drugs, alcohol or cigarettes, learning to function without any sex at all is not possible when trying to build or maintain an intimate relationship.

Understanding how a healthy sexual and intimate relationship looks and feels can be difficult after sexual addiction treatment. As a child abuse survivor, recovered sex addict, and therapist, Maureen Canning speaks from experience as she identifies the 10 characteristics of a healthy relationship in her book *Lust, Anger, Love: Understanding Sexual Addiction and the Road to Healthy Intimacy.*

1. **Sex provides a feeling of wellbeing.**
   There is a safety in a healthy relationship that may be a bit

scary at first. It will take patience and perseverance to move beyond the feelings of disconnection and shame that may have been part of the previous sexual experiences.

2. **Emotional and physical sensations are more positive.**
   Romantic intimacy requires vulnerability and emotional honesty without numbing or "chasing the orgasm."

3. **Creativity and passion are rediscovered.**
   As sex is no longer the only outlet for emotional expression, the brain learns to use these tools for creative exploration in new ways.

4. **You nurture yourself in non-genital ways.**
   Pleasure is expanded beyond the previously exclusive channel of sexuality to include all aspects of life.

5. **Suffering is tolerated as a part of life.**
   When life's challenges, disappointments, and difficulties come along, they are dealt with in a more cerebral rather than sexual way. They are faced, not hidden.

6. **You can be emotionally vulnerable.**
   It is common for sexual addicts to fear betrayal and to suppress their feelings instead of risk being hurt. In a healthy relationship, vulnerability is not only acceptable but also necessary.

7. **You develop and maintain healthy boundaries with others.**
   Boundaries are the enemy for many addicts and in some cases work as the trigger for destructive behavior. Acknowledging, accepting and embracing the safety within these romantic boundaries are an important part of recovery.

8. **Sexuality is well balanced and moderate.**
   Sexual energy in all its extremes is used to motivate the life of a sex addict. With sexual maturity comes the appropriate flow of this energy.

9. **You are curious and caring about other people's reactions to you.**
   Whereas sex addiction is very ego-driven and the emotional lives of others are kept at a distance, healthy intimacy requires empathy and understanding for your partner's point of view.

10. **You learn to trust others.**
    The first step in overcoming sexual addiction is learning to trust yourself and accepting the truth of who you are. This personal trust gives you the courage to lower your guard enough to invite in the truth and trust of a partner.

Breaking Up Is Hard To Do

Sadly, the best intentions, hardest work, and most earnest dedication can't save every relationship. I will, of course, tell you that every ending holds the seeds of a new beginning, but who wants to hear about that when you're in the middle of a horrible break up or divorce?

Break ups can involve the full scope of ugly emotions including anger, anxiety, depression, and loneliness. Recovery isn't fast either. A study performed by biological anthropologist Helen Fisher shows that 40% of people still exhibit signs of clinical depression eight weeks after the end of a romantic relationship. This prolonged emotional reaction isn't a sign of evolutionary weakness, either. Instead it's a primitive response rooted in the social bonding that helps the species survive and reproduce.

The way in which a partner is attached will determine how the breakup is processed psychologically. Like many of the scales associated with a person's personality make-up (left brain to right brain, extroversion, Kinsey's Heterosexual-Homosexual Rating Scale), there also exists a spectrum of attachment styles. At one end is anxious attachment, defined by extreme neediness and insecurity. The other end of the scale is represented by avoidant attachment that eludes commitment and openness. As you can imagine, the anxious partners will be most challenged by a breakup and are more likely to turn to unhealthy coping mechanisms, such as drinking, while the avoiders will have a much easier time moving on.

Though stereotypes may lead you to think that women are more likely to have difficulty with the end of a relationship, this isn't necessarily true. Given two-thirds of divorces are instigated by women and the fact that their emotional intelligence is more finely tuned to register relationship warning signs, the female population actually holds the upper hand.

To learn how the brain responds to a break up, Dr. Helen Fisher performed an MRI scan while participants looked at pictures of the ex-partners who had recently ended their relationship. Several regions of the brain showed increased activity, especially those associated with motivation, addiction, obsessive-compulsive disorder and reward.

By triggering the reward center, the pleasure hormone of dopamine is released in anticipation of seeing this loved one. As the brain realizes that the ex won't be coming, this reward center becomes deprived, waking up the middle part of the brain, namely the ventral tegmental area (VTA) and nucleus accumbens. As these two areas analyze the pluses and minuses of this ended relationship, the nearby prefrontal cortex triggers the emotions of frustration and anger.

If that's not brutal enough, the brain also interprets the pain of a breakup in the same way it reads the burn of a flame. Neurologists at the Einstein College of Medicine found that seeing photographs of ex-partners

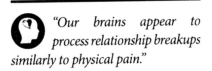

"*Our brains appear to process relationship breakups similarly to physical pain.*"

– Dr. Melanie Greenberg

ignited the same brain region that processes physical discomfort and releases the stress hormone cortisol. And if you've ever felt like trying to get over an ex was like trying to break an awful addiction, you're literally correct. Another test by Dr. Fisher found that the brain of someone recovering from a break up looks eerily similar to the brain scan of someone working to overcome a cocaine addiction.

After that barrage of uncomfortable information, let me boldly state that, regardless of how it may feel in the moment, breakups can inspire incredible, positive life changes. I do not believe that you are given one true love in life. And even if you are, why would it be the person that didn't want to stay with you?

Moving on isn't easy when you have to rediscover the world as a "me" instead of a "we" but it has the potential to be a truly extraordinary adventure. It's necessary to grieve the loss of a relationship but it's equally necessary to keep moving forward. Make plans. Spring clean. Take a trip. Give a Break-Up party. As John Lennon is credited with saying, "Everything is okay in the end. If it's not okay, then it's not the end." Your saga is still unfolding; so don't confuse the end of a chapter for the end of your story.

An Open Mind And An Open Heart

There's a lot of darkness that can come through life but it's only because of this dark that we learn to appreciate the light. The internal work we do to understand our own minds gives us the tools and the foundation to create an ever better external life, and this most definitely applies to our romantic relationships. The more clearly we see ourselves, the more we are able to see and embrace the ones we love. Regardless of the circumstances life hands out, there is peace and joy and comfort to be found as long as there is a commitment to make happiness a priority. Like the first Prime Minister of India, Jawaharlal Nehru, stated, "Life is like a game of cards. The hand you are dealt is determinism; the way you play it is free will." Keep reading for some insight into maintaining a winning hand while Playing The Cards We're Dealt.

CHAPTER NINE
Playing The Cards We're Dealt

Just like break-ups, sometimes unpleasant things happen in life and we are forced to play the cards we're dealt. A chronic illness, a physical disability, a traumatic event beyond our control – there are some things that are just no fun. But life also gives us choices, and we can certainly choose how we react to these events, allowing them to build our strength and character, or letting them doom us to eternal suffering. Which would you choose?

I was so relieved when my husband promised to tell me if anyone ever threatened him physically again, and even more relieved when he increased the security around our home. Emotionally, I was feeling quite "over" the violent attack against him, but my body took a different path. I began to have acute pain in the right side of my face, ear, jaw and teeth. Twelve root canals later I still had the pain and it was only becoming more acute. I was next diagnosed with TMJ (Tempro Mandibular Joint Syndrome), a misalignment of the teeth and/or jaw, which can cause excruciating pain and migraine headaches. The pain had become piercing, almost constant and felt as if an ice pick was being jammed into my jaw. Often the condition was so debilitating that it was impossible for me to sleep, and after trying many different treatments I was still no better.

As a last resort, I had MRI and Cat scan tests done to see if I had any neurological problems. I was diagnosed with Trigeminal Neuralgia (TGN), a condition involving a blood vessel pressing against a nerve in my brain. My physicians recommended brain surgery and convinced me that my condition was not going to go into remission, so, when my husband asked me what I wanted for Christmas, I didn't hesitate to answer, "Brain surgery!" I could think of no greater present than to be rid of the maddening pain I was in. Peter agreed that I should have the endoscopic micro neuro-decompression surgery.

Well, that was in January 2000 and even though the surgery was not a success, I had another surgery a few months later called The Gama Knife that didn't help either. I was prescribed a myriad of medications that had no effect, and now I have finally learned to live with the pain in the hopes that one day it will disappear as fast as it appeared.

I believe that it was triggered by the shock of seeing my husband bleeding to death with his neck cut from ear to ear. It was a nightmare, but I couldn't scream. Instead I did everything I could to save his life, and I'm so very grateful that worked, but my body is paying a price.

This physical misfortune has opened my eyes even wider to human vulnerability. I realize how minor my problem is in relation to the suffering of others, and it makes me want to help people even more.

I now view challenges as coming complete with their own inherent solutions. Every situation that crosses our path is a gift, but not every gift comes in a cheerful package. It is how we perceive the gift, and what we do with it, that counts. One of the gifts of my profound trauma and subsequent physical pain is that it activated my interest in neuroscience, which led me to writing this book.

Intimacy After Illness

One situation that makes it difficult to find a silver lining is facing illness. Just consider the top five medical threats: heart disease, cancer, stroke, chronic respiratory diseases, and Alzheimer's disease. Not exactly a happy list, right? Anyone who

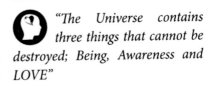

"The Universe contains three things that cannot be destroyed; Being, Awareness and LOVE"

– Dr. Deepak Chopra

has suffered from illness knows that feeling of helplessness and fear of a future without intimacy. Maintaining positive mental health can be a tremendous aid in dealing with challenges like this. In fact, while your fears about your partner's illness may compel you to push away the person you love the most, this could be an opportunity to enhance intimacy.

Most couples that really love each other discover that their love grows stronger and their passion deeper after trauma because they no longer take each other for granted. They fall back in love and want to treasure every moment. This is the time to start re-creating romantic memories together, to say and do all the things you did when you first met and some you never did before.

Rabbi Ed Weinberg, Ed.D., DD, offers a lot of great insight into overcoming illness and recapturing your intimacy in his book, *Conquer Prostate Cancer: How Medicine, Faith, Love and Sex Can Renew Your Life.* Guided by Rabbi Ed's heart-centered coaching, men and women learn to reignite intimacy physically, emotionally and spiritually — loving and living with renewed joy. He believes that physical intimacy can help a man or woman offset some of their frustrations when one or both have a sexual dysfunction that prevents intercourse or orgasm.

It's my pleasure to share Rabbi Ed's advice on how you and your partner can get your sexual life back despite prostate cancer.

NEURO-CISE: S.T.I.C.K, DUO

1. Decide to "make love," rather than "have sex."

Physical intimacy can help a man or woman offset some of their frustrations when one or both have a sexual dysfunction that prevents intercourse or orgasm. To offset this, recognize that orgasm is possible for many, although not everyone, even when men can't have erections due to ED or women have female sexual dysfunctions (FSD).

Don't insist that your manhood is exclusively based on your capacity for intercourse. Instead of sexual intercourse, make bonding with your partner your main objective. It's understandable that losing sexual functioning can lead to a sense of emasculation as a man or deficiency as a woman. Still, if you accept that "making love" rather than "having sex" is at the core of your most intimate moments, you may find increasing sexual satisfaction. This is not a question of semantics, but a way to reframe what intimacy is all about.

2. Focus on different body sensations before engaging in intercourse, using the S-T-I-C-K method for "whole body sex."

This is a variation of progressive "sensate focus" for gradually increasing arousal. Couples may choose to alternate this suggested sequence of sensual activities or combine some of these steps:

S - Stroke each other psychologically. Almost everyone needs to be stroked. Start with verbal expressions of what you admire most about each other and what attracts you to each other intellectually, spiritually, emotionally, and physically.

T - Touch each other physically, starting with a hug, whether clothed or not. Proceed to mutual massages, front and back, gradually progressing from your shoulders to your waist, avoiding your partner's breasts. Then proceed to touch or massage each other's legs before gently caressing erogenous zones like each other's breasts, thighs and genitals.

I - Intercourse can be attempted right after stroking and touching, or later if you are "up" for it – but don't rush it! Many men, including early stage and advanced prostate or breast cancer patients and survivors, may find their sexual frustration persists despite the satisfaction they can derive from whole body alternative sex play. If ED or FSD persists, the couple can consider a soft entry approach, with the man's flaccid penis rubbing the surface of his partner's genitalia. Using a dildo and harness can also be mutually satisfying, and if both partners apply lubrication both men and women can make this a more pleasant and pleasurable experience. A penile implant, requiring about 1 1/2 hours of surgery, is another option for men to eliminate ED altogether.

C - Cuddle without initial expectations of anything but deriving warmth and support, physically and emotionally.

K - Kiss each other gently on the lips, cheeks, and back. Then go below the neck, but above the waist. From there, your lips can go elsewhere, if mutually acceptable (compare "T"). Adding a mixture of whipped cream or your favorite chocolate can heighten your pleasure.

3. Communicate openly and often with your spouse or partner.
Be truly present when talking with your beloved about non-sexual matters. After all, you can have smooth, ongoing relations only if you have a good relationship! Set aside time to talk with your spouse or partner about your personal needs, especially sexual intimacy. If talking explicitly about sex is awkward for either of you, you can each write down what you need or want from each other and then compare notes and follow up.

Explore alternatives as well like tantric sex exercises, originally derived from 6,000 year-old Indian practices that help lovers focus on each other for a prolonged time. This involves mutual eye contact and parallel movement and breathing, to become fully present and at one with each other and potentially multi-orgasmic. Attending a Marriage Enrichment weekend retreat can also reinforce your connection with your significant other on many levels.

4. Schedule times to rev up your romance.

Sexual relations are hard to sustain without developing a good relationship. Set dates with each other to allow for greater non-sexual intimacy, such as seeing a movie or going to a restaurant or concert together. Use scented candles and wear special pajamas or lingerie (or nothing at all!) with soft lighting, to set the mood for increased physical intimacy.

5. Watch a hot movie together that appeals to your sense of humor.

Agree to rent a steamy film for home or hotel room viewing to help get you and your partner in the mood to become physical. Make sure you do not choose a film that is going to turn one of you on, but the other off, and remember that a humorous show can warm you up to each other! Keep in mind that some educational films, though approved by sexologists, may be boring and fail to arouse couples, so preview films to see what works best for you.

6. Develop a healthy lifestyle.

Exercise regularly and eat a balanced, heart-healthy, low-sugar diet for weight control and improved sleep. Reduce alcohol intake to avoid sluggishness and eliminate smoking to enhance genital blood flow. Such steps can renew your level of energy and reduce performance anxiety. Let your mantra be, "I enjoy my sexercises" to maintain penile or vaginal blood flow through self or mutual-stimulation. Start this as soon as possible after a health procedure such as cancer surgery or other procedures, in consultation with your doctor.

Daily Kegel exercises, with the help of biofeedback if needed, can strengthen your pelvic floor and sphincter muscles. While these won't raise your libido, Kegels can help with ED and FSD. They will also help "stem the tide" for those with mild incontinence.

7. Keep the faith.

To conquer ED or FSD and raise your libido, have faith in your Higher Power, your doctor, your spouse, and above all, yourself. Regarding sexual activity as sacred or purposeful can make for a more powerful experience.

It's important to recognize that stress, treatment side effects, and the aging process can affect not only seniors but boomers and younger men and women as well. Simply knowing you are not alone in your efforts to renew your life physically, emotionally and spiritually can help. It's equally important, though, to realize that you can bounce back from ED/FSD and a low libido if you resolve to rely on your resilience and your adaptability to new forms of sexual expression. This kind of faith can raise you to new heights!

With over 280,000 new cases of breast cancer each year in the United States, there are over 2.5 million survivors of breast cancer. According to the National Cancer Institute, about one out of every two women who have undergone breast cancer treatment experiences some kind of sexual dysfunction.

When a woman has a mastectomy to remove all or part of her breast(s), her body may be capable of sexual response, but sexual desire is one of the last things on her mind. It's no surprise that many women feel very distressed after a mastectomy as in our culture breasts are viewed as part of a woman's femininity and sex appeal. Not to mention that touching breasts is a common part of foreplay and she will no longer want or be able to experience the same way as before the surgery. Breast reconstruction may restore the shape and size of the breast(s) and help a woman to feel more attractive so that she can enjoy dating or being sexual with her partner, but the physical and emotional healing process is much bigger than a simple cosmetic fix and requires a tremendous amount of time, understanding and respect.

Being single and dating when diagnosed with breast cancer is even more challenging as talking about it to a potential romantic partner can be very awkward and scary. Nevertheless, getting out and socializing is part of the healing process and will help you to feel normal again. There is a fine balance that needs to be walked between respecting your own needs while also trying to push yourself a bit beyond your comfort level in order to reengage with the world. Small steps are important because even the smallest connection with another person can aid the healing process.

According to the American Breast Cancer Society, breast cancer is about 100 times less common among men than women. For men, the lifetime risk of getting breast cancer is about 1 in 1,000 compared to women at about 1 in 8. Twelve percent of women in the U.S. will develop invasive breast cancer during their lifetime.

Undergoing extensive treatment from surgery to medication, chemotherapy or radiation can be detrimental to your sexiness. Stress, anxiety, changes in body image, side effects of treatment, pain, hormone fluctuations and depression can negatively affect your libido. However, the good news is that you can heal and regain your sexual health.

Research by Barry Komisaruk, Beverly Whipple ("The Science of Orgasm") and their colleagues has shown that women with complete spinal cord injury can respond to vaginal or cervical self-stimulation because they could perceive it, with some reporting an orgasmic response. A spinal cord injury, traumatic brain injury, or major illness does not diminish a person's sexuality, although it may change a person's feeling about sex.

Intimate communication with your partner can be challenging, but remember nobody can read your mind, so tell each other what is working and what isn't. Being direct with other people helps the relationship grow. However, some people who have intellectual or physical disabilities may find it hard to express their anxieties about body image or limited sexual function. Show your personality and humor during these uncomfortable moments because laughter can make the situation more comfortable.

If there is an inability to experience sexual release, some say that sexual energy can be moved up into the mind. Channel, build, utilize and move the energy into having a mental orgasm. Start by visualizing the orgasmic flow inside you, knowing that orgasm is within and focus on erotic feelings that lead to physical tingling orgasmic waves as they pulse through your body. There has been some scientific research on energy orgasms. Most notably, Dr. Beverly Whipple calls it "Thinking Off" and says that you can use imagery alone to reach an orgasm, but the idea of thinking yourself to orgasm is not new. In the early 1970's, the Masters and Johnson research team documented the strong connection between sexuality and thought. The connection is particularly strong in women, says Dr. Ian Kerner, "The brain is the most powerful sex organ."

NEURO-CISE: SEXUAL HEALING, SOLO

With the understanding that each individual is different, here are 10 steps to help get your sexy back.

1. **Reach Out**
   Different people experience varying levels of physical, mental and social anguish, but it is important to remember that there is hope. If you have a lack of desire from a hormone imbalance, issues with body image or just a lack of support and understanding, it may contribute to social withdrawal, canceling plans with friends, shying away from family functions, etc. Reaching out is key to improving the whole person on the inside and the outside.

2. **Define Your True Self**
   The first step in improving relationships with others is to take an inward look at yourself to build self-confidence and self-esteem. If you're single and not dating anyone special, there's no need to immediately share your medical history or disclose your cancer. Be sure to let your date see all of your healthy qualities, fun attributes and fabulous personality. Then see if there is any relationship possibility before you disclose your prognosis, as you do not want to define yourself by your physical condition.

3. Feel Heard

The best way to clear feelings of fear, guilt, insecurity or even neglect is through open and honest communication. I know it's not always easy to ask for what you want; so one way to start is to ask for little things, like a hug. Then let your partner know where you are emotionally by telling them explicitly with no-holds-barred honesty. One of the fundamentals to accessing your sexiness and letting go of inhibitions is feeling heard. Provide open communication about your needs to help make you feel sexy again, even if it is just patience!

4. Monitor Your Libido

It's a fact that some medications and treatments that help to fight illness have side effects that can diminish your libido. Monitoring what time of day or night you feel most energetic or more relaxed can help you tap into your own comfort level with regards to romance or sexuality. A vital part of getting your sexy back is to know yourself so that you can better share that inner sexpot with your partner.

5. Laugh Your Way to Health

Humor and playfulness with friends, family, dates or lovers can trigger positive thoughts and emotional connections. Laughter is also a powerful remedy for pain, stress, depression and whatever ails you as it releases feel-good hormones and prompts healthy changes in the body. Watch comedies on TV, at the movies or share jokes and funny stories to experience the healing power of laughter as it improves your mental, emotional and physical health. In my seminars for couples I always ask them to share the funniest moment in their relationship as an interactive exercise that helps to make them feel close.

6. Build Your Strength

Physical exercises can help to reduce the risk of many health risks and help people to feel better while going through treatments. A balance of aerobic, strength training and stretching is important, but always check with your doctor before undergoing any strenuous exercise regimen. Do your Kegel exercises regularly to strengthen the sexual muscles, and especially right before intercourse to get the blood flowing to your genitals.

7. **Create Your Own Shangri-La**
Remove yourself from reality and create your own sensory escapism-like Shangri-La, a place of paradise and bliss. Light the bathroom with candles, put on soothing music, and fill the tub with bubbles, warm water and flower petals. Enjoy the way you feel. Release yourself from negative thoughts and worries. Focus on the delight of eating some of your favorite foods such as chocolates or ice cream and get into a sexy state of mind by enhancing all five of your senses. Surrender to the pleasures of your own personal Shangri-La.

8. **Connect Through Healing Touch**
Especially during trying times, couples need to communicate their needs, so tell your partner that a healing massage would be a great way to relieve tension, improve blood circulation and relax your mind and body. Tell your partner the places you would like to be massaged the most. Massage is a mutually satisfying way of helping couples to exhibit intimacy for one another. It is a precious gift that you can give to your partner when they need it most.

9. **Use Enhancers and Enablers**
Essential oils with jasmine, rosemary, and sage are said to increase arousal when rubbed on the skin. Applying them to erogenous zones like the neck and to stress-carrying areas like the back and shoulders can stir sensuous feelings. For intimate dryness, be sure to have some personal lubricant ready to make sexual intercourse more comfortable and reduce friction or discomfort. Lubricants can also enhance masturbation for a smoother, silkier and wetter solo-sexual experience.

10. **Practice Brain Sex**

The brain is the largest sex organ in the body so maintaining an optimistic outlook goes a long way to supporting and rebuilding a healthy sex life. Sexiness encompasses much more than intercourse. As mentioned above, communication, laughter, setting the mood, healing touch, giving yourself permission to surrender and getting yourself into a juicy state of mind are all key elements to getting your sexy back.

Cardio Loveology

There is a misconception that heart disease is a man's disease when, according to the American Heart Association (AHA), heart disease, it is the leading cause of death for American women. Some patients give up having sex

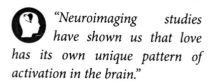

"Neuroimaging studies have shown us that love has its own unique pattern of activation in the brain."

– Kayt Sukel

after a heart attack for fear of another heart attack, and they're too embarrassed to talk to their doctor about it.

The emotional heart can take longer to heal than the physical heart in the sense that many patients feel frail after coming so close to death. They put sex on hold, not realizing that abstinence can lead to depression and seriously affect the quality of a relationship. Some cardiologists recommend resuming sexual activity when their patients can climb up a couple of flights of stairs without getting out of breath, while others prescribe an exercise stress test to check how much physical activity the heart can handle with ease. Many experts also advise waiting from one to three hours after eating a big meal to allow for digestion. "Think of sex as a particularly enjoyable workout," Dr. Wayne Sotile writes in his book, *Thriving with Heart Disease*. He advises heart attack patients to pace themselves and ease back into sexual activity.

It's also best to try to have sex only when you feel rested and relaxed.

"Don't forget the relationship aspect of it," Dr. Sotile says. "To the extent that your relationship is comfortable, you will be relaxed and you will much more likely be able to function sexually."

"Heart disease gives you a second chance. Most of us in long-term relationships could use some do-overs," he adds. "I encourage people to respond to the wake-up call that heart disease delivers to make your life better." Many heart attack survivors have told Sotile that they've become more "caring, loving and patient" after their heart attacks.

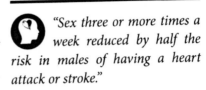

"Sex three or more times a week reduced by half the risk in males of having a heart attack or stroke."

- Dr. Daniel G. Amen

After a heart attack, recovery is different for everyone and the more love you give yourself, the quicker your emotional heart will heal. One easy way to love yourself is to give yourself a gentle heart-hug by putting your hand on your heart and feel the sense of security as your brain releases oxytocin and reduces anxiety to make way for loving thoughts.

NEURO-CISE: HEART HEALING, SOLO

Linda Graham, author of *Bouncing Back: Rewiring Your Brain for Maximum Resilience and Wellbeing*, offers experiential exercises of "self-directed neuroplasticity" and has over eighty exercises in her book that allow you to do this rewiring safely, efficiently and effectively. Her "Hand on the Heart" exercise is much more profound than the heart hug.

1. Begin by placing your hand on your heart, feeling the warmth of your own touch. Breathe gently and deeply into your heart center, taking in a sense of calm, peace, goodness, safety, trust, acceptance, and ease.

2. Once that's steady, call to mind a moment of being with

someone who loves you unconditionally, someone you feel completely safe with. This may, of course, be a partner, child, or parent; but if the dynamics of those relationships are complicated and the emotions mixed, you may choose any true other to your true self: a dear friend, a trusted teacher, a close colleague or neighbor, a therapist, your grandmother, a spiritual figure like Jesus or the Dalai Lama, or your wiser self. Pets are also great for this exercise.

3. As you remember feeling safe and loved with this person or pet, see if you can sense in your body the positive feelings and sensations associated with that memory. Really savor a feeling of warmth, safety, trust, and love in your body.

4. When that feeling is steady, let go of the image and simply bathe in the feeling itself for thirty seconds. Savor the rich nurturing of this feeling; let it really soak in.

Breathing deeply, gently, and fully activates the calming branch of our autonomic nervous system, the parasympathetic branch. The parasympathetic modulates the brain's fight-flight-freeze response when we feel threatened or agitated. Breathing, or pranayama, has been a core practice in yoga and meditation to relax the body and steady the mind for over 3,500 years.

Breathing positive emotions into the heart center steadies the heart rate, restoring the equilibrium of the body so that we can remain present and engaged. In recalling a memory or image of feeling loved and cherished, we evoke a sense of safe connection with others; the oxytocin immediately reduces our stress. That evocation also activates the prefrontal cortex, which triggers the hippocampus to search for explicit memories of moments when we have been held, soothed, protected, encouraged, believed in, times when we have reached out for help and received comfort and support.

Through safety and trust in connection, we come back into our baseline equilibrium. From there, with our higher, thinking brain calm and alert, we can mobilize quickly, act skillfully, and take care of business.

How to Have Sex with A, B and C

Arthritis, Back and Chronic Pain all have a significant impact on daily activities and the general enjoyment of life. The National Institute of Arthritis and Musculoskeletal and Skin Diseases reports that eight out of ten Americans will suffer from back pain at some point in their lives. So if you or your partner has arthritis, back pain or any kind of chronic pain, then it's not surprising that your sex life is limited.

A new review by The National Center for Complementary and Alternative Medicine (NCCAM) researchers in *Nature Reviews Neuroscience* looks at recent research on pain and the brain. It suggests that chronic pain affects the anatomy of the brain and impairs certain nerve pathways, leading to a "negative feedback loop" that results in more pain and accompanying emotional and reasoning problems. What's exciting about this discovery is that feedback loops can be mitigated by mindful meditation. Many people affected by chronic pain are learning how the mind can control the body, and are adopting practices such as meditation and yoga to reduce stress and control pain.

Dr. Rick Hanson, a neuropsychologist and author of *Buddha's Brain: The Practical Neuroscience of Happiness, Love and Wisdom* says, "One of the enduring changes in the brain of those who routinely meditate is that the brain becomes thicker. In other words, those who routinely meditate build synapses, synaptic networks, and layers of capillaries (the tiny blood vessels that bring metabolic supplies such as glucose or oxygen to busy regions), which an MRI shows is measurably thicker in two major regions of the brain. One is in the pre-frontal cortex, located right behind the forehead. It's involved in the executive control of attention – of deliberately paying attention to something. This change makes sense because that's what you're doing when you meditate or engage in a contemplative activity. The second brain area that gets bigger is a very important part called the insula. The insula tracks both the interior state of the body and the feelings of other people, which is fundamental to empathy. So, people who routinely tune into their own bodies – through some kind of mindfulness practice – make their insula thicker, which helps them become more self-aware and empathic." This is a good illustration of "neuroplasticity," which is the idea that "as the mind changes, the brain changes," or as Canadian psychologist Donald Hebb puts it, "neurons that fire together wire together."

In her book, *A Slice of the Beloved,* Gurutej Kaur shares her forty years of yoga teachings, with exercises for singles and couples that can heal the mind and the body.

NEURO-CISE: HAND DUSTING, SOLO

Quickly and powerfully move your hands, in front of your heart center, as if dusting them off. This will help bring calm and quiet. It is also great way to release a distressing thought or experience.

NEURO-CISE: CONNECTION MEDITATION, DUO

Sit across from each other on your heels or in a comfortable pose. Lean forward, placing your foreheads together. Place your hands on each other's shoulders or around the waist. This posture connects third eye to third-eye, stimulating the pituitary gland and intuition spot.

Talk It Through

Equally important to exercise is good communication with your partner. He or she cannot help you or create a better lovemaking experience if you don't share the experience of your pain. Sharing a warm bath and experimenting with pillows can be a way to relax and begin the process towards intimacy.

"Talk about it," says Ian Kerner, a sexuality counselor and author of *She Comes First: The Thinking Man's Guide to Pleasing a Woman.* "Back pain can be tricky because people often look fine, even if they feel terrible. That's all the more reason to keep your partner in the loop. Don't try to please your partner at the expense of hurting yourself. Your partner will feel the distraction in your body language, and conclude that something is wrong. If you're not forthcoming that the 'something' is back pain, their imagination could run wild."

Joint pain can make sexual contact uncomfortable, but don't give up trying new positions or timing of sexual activity. There may be certain positions that would work better than others, to bring you both satisfaction without one person having to "grin and bear it."

It can feel awkward at first to talk to your partner about how you're going to make love, but you may find that the experience deepens your connection with each other. The steps taken to find comfortable sexual positions such as Spooning or Scissors can bring you back to the same page, erotically speaking.

If your pain is much too severe to try having sex, talk to a medical professional and take solace in the fact that the severity is likely temporary, and focus on other acts that can maintain your intimacy without rigorous performance. Get comfortable and hold hands, then start kissing and enjoy locking lips for as long as you can.

Sheril Kirshenbaum, author of *The Science of Kissing: What Our Lips Are Telling Us*, writes, "The part of our bodies sending the most information to our brains during a kiss is, without a doubt, the lips. Packed with nerve endings, they are extremely sensitive to pressure, warmth, cold, and indeed to every kind of stimulus. One of the most remarkable things about the brain's role in kissing is the disproportionate neural space associated with our lips compared with the rest of our bodies. Just a light brush on them stimulates a very large part of the brain - an area even more expansive than would be activated by sexual stimulation below the belt. A kiss sends sensations directly to the limbic system that part of our brain associated with love, passion, and lust. As neural impulses bounce between the brain and the tongue, the facial muscles, the lips, and the skin, they stimulate our bodies to produce a number of neurotransmitters and hormones."

Menopause and Andropause

Another hand we're dealt as human beings is getting older, and that comes with physical changes like hormonal shifts. You're probably all thinking about menopause, but changes in hormones are not exclusively a female issue. It's a natural part of aging that affects both sexes, though for men the changes happen more gradually while women tend to experience a dramatic hormone plunge. In women, ovulation ends and hormone production plummets during a relatively short period of time.

Often referred to as "andropause," men can experience a decrease in testosterone, sexual function, energy and mood swings but these changes may be subtle and can go unnoticed for years.

Symptoms of decreased testosterone may include:

- ♥ Changes in sexual function, including erectile dysfunction, reduced sexual desire, and infertility. Testes might become smaller as well.

- ♥ Changes in sleep patterns, either with insomnia or increased fatigue.

- ♥ Physical changes such as increased body fat, reduced muscle mass and strength, and decreased bone density, sensitive breasts (gynecomastia), and body hair loss.

- ♥ Emotional changes such as decreased motivation or self-confidence and increased bouts of depression.

- ♥ Trouble concentrating or remembering things.

- ♥ Though far more likely in women going through menopause, it is also possible for men to experience hot flashes.

As all of these symptoms can indicate other ailments such as thyroid problems or medication side effects, a blood test is the only way to properly diagnose a decrease in testosterone.

Though the prospect of aging and menopause is often met with trepidation and depression in many women, Dr. Louann Brizendine and author of *The Female Brain*, argues "the change will set you free." For the 150,000 women who enter menopause each month in America alone, this may be revolutionary news. As Dr. Brizendine sees it, the decline in hormones that comes with menopause allows for a whole new approach to life that can be equal parts confusing and liberating.

Fundamentally, menopause marks the end of the "mommy brain" that had previously put a higher focus on the needs of others, especially children and romantic partners. As the ebb and flow of estrogen and progesterone levels out, the call to be a caretaker decreases as the production of oxytocin declines sharply. Dr. Brizendine points out that the "estrogenized brain" is more wired to be nurturing and protective of our relationships. However, menopause causes a decrease in estrogen, which places the level closer to that of the amount of testosterone women carry. These new hormone levels makes a woman's brain more like a man's so she may become more prone to anger or, at the very least, less likely to embrace a path of passivity.

These changes have great potential to create conflict in romantic relationships because there can be tremendous shifts in how a woman reacts to situations, and how she perceives her role in a partnership. She may be more prone to angry outbursts and less able to overlook things when they disappoint, aggravate or offend her. According to Dr. Brizendine, after the age of menopause, 65% of divorces are initiated by women, pointing to the dramatic shift in what they are willing to tolerate after these hormonal changes finally settle down.

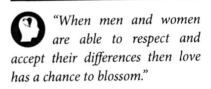

"When men and women are able to respect and accept their differences then love has a chance to blossom."

– *Dr. John Gray*

Aging Is An Honor

The brain itself goes through some changes over the course of a lifetime as well. The Dana Foundation is a private philanthropic organization committed to advancing brain research and to educating the public on the scientific discoveries of how the brain works. In their extensive reference guide, *The Dana Guide to Brain Health*, their team of medical experts dedicates a lot of time to how the brain evolves over the course of a lifetime. About the aging process, they state, "The most important trait the brain brings to adulthood and through the end of life can be summed up in one word, "plasticity."

Neuroscientists created the term plasticity to define the brain's biological evolution when confronted with new experiences or change. This is how we learn, develop, and break habits, adjust to new situations and surroundings, and cope with surprises, changes, challenges, and opportunities that make up the process of living. Without this plasticity, every new encounter would remain scary and uncertain.

As age progresses, the thick bundle of nerve fibers known as the corpus callosum decrease in size. It is through these fibers that the two halves of the brain pass messages, so this would create a delay in what might have previously been an immediate response. Additionally, the ability to quickly, easily and coherently shift focus from one task or idea to another begins to weaken, starting at middle age, which can lead to a response of irritability toward distractions that used to be more easily managed.

 "The brain is primed to focus on what changes, rather than what remains in a steady state."

– Sandra J. Ackerman

Also, the ability to choose NOT to pay attention to something we consider unimportant — a ticking clock, a neighbor's loud party, the drip of a leaky faucet — is not a skill we are born with, but one that we learn in early development and it begins to weaken later in life, which can add to a sense of being easily distracted.

As the scientific and medical fields have begun to properly diagnose people with Alzheimer's disease, the concept of senility being a part of the aging process has slowly gone away. While the speed with which things can be done both mentally and physically may be slowed down a bit, a majority of brain functions remain intact throughout a lifetime. Just because your body may not work well on the outside doesn't mean that it won't work well on the inside.

Allow yourself to appreciate, relax, relish and accept pleasant experiences. Start saying "yes" to more positive moments and "no" to people making demands on your valuable time, as it's the most precious gift to give to yourself. Know that a disability or chronic illness does not equal a disabled sex drive.

NEURO-CISE: STAYING YOUTHFUL, SOLO

While some aspects of aging can't be controlled, there are many things that will help ensure a longer life, both mentally and physically. The Harvard Medical School offers twelve ways to help your brain retain its power.

1. **Get mental stimulation.**
   Like any other muscle in the body, the brain only stays strong if it's being used and challenged regularly. Learn a new skill, read about interesting topics, and work on puzzles that require concentration, do craftwork that requires dexterity such as drawing or painting. Create a scrapbook of your relationship or create the love life that you want to manifest with pictures.

2. **Get physical exercise.**
   Exercise inspires the development of new nerve cells and increases the synapses between brain cells. This supports an efficient, flexible and adaptive brain while also creating a host of health benefits, such as lower blood pressure, improved cholesterol levels, and reduction in mental stress. Kiss the left side of your partner's body to stimulate the right side of their brain. Hold hands using your non-dominant hand to

trigger the opposite side of the brain. Sexual activity is a great workout for your pelvic floor muscles and orgasms cause contractions that also strengthen them.

3. **Improve your diet.**
   Nutrition is as important to a healthy brain as it is to a healthy body. A reduced caloric intake has been shown to lower the risk of mental decline. Not only do you need to eat LESS you also need to eat BETTER by reducing the consumption of saturated fat and cholesterol from animal sources and of trans-fatty acids from partially hydrogenated vegetable oils. Dementia has been linked to high levels of homocysteine, which can be reduced by increasing your intake of the three B vitamins, folic acid, B6, and B12. Fortified cereal, other grains, and leafy green vegetables are good sources of B vitamins. Feed each other phallic looking vegetables and fruits to boost your health and your libido at the same time.

4. **Improve your blood pressure.**
   High blood pressure in midlife increases the risk of cognitive decline in old age. Many of the ideas outlined in this list help control blood pressure, so stay lean, exercise regularly, limit your alcohol to two drinks a day, reduce stress, and eat right. Research suggests a link between sex and lower blood pressure, says Joseph J. Pinzone, MD. He is CEO and medical director of Amai Wellness. "One landmark study found that sexual intercourse specifically (not masturbation) lowered systolic blood pressure."

5. **Improve your blood sugar.**
   Diabetes is an important risk factor for dementia. You can fight diabetes by eating right, exercising regularly, and staying lean. But if your blood sugar stays high, you'll need medication to achieve good control.

6. **Improve your cholesterol.**
   High levels of LDL ("bad") cholesterol increase the risk of

dementia, as do low levels of HDL ("good") cholesterol. Diet, exercise, weight control, and avoiding tobacco will go a long way toward improving your cholesterol levels. But if you need more help, ask your doctor about medication.

7. **Consider low-dose aspirin.**
Observational studies suggest that long-term use of aspirin and other nonsteroidal anti-inflammatory drugs (NSAIDs) may reduce the risk of dementia by 10%–55%. It's hopeful information, but it's preliminary. Experts are not ready to recommend aspirin specifically for dementia.

8. **Avoid tobacco.**
I can't imagine you need me to explain this in any greater detail, but you might not know that smoking makes the taste of your body's juices turn bitter. Quit smoking, and you'll live longer and taste better. Enough said.

9. **Don't abuse alcohol.**
Alcoholic intake is an interesting balancing act because excessive drinking has been linked to dementia while moderate drinking has been shown to reduce the risk of dementia. It is recommended that if you are going to drink, that you limit yourself to two drinks a day. According to the National Institute of Health, alcohol increases the risks of sexual dysfunction and can affect one's abilities in the bedroom. Not only that, but too much booze can cloud your judgment and increase the likelihood of having unprotected sex.

10. **Care for your emotions.**
Mental health and restful sleep are important tools in maintaining cognition. Taking the necessary steps to reduce and fight anxiety, depression, and exhaustion can go a long way toward supporting long time mental fortitude. If you're single, make sure that you have control of your emotions before you have sex with a new partner.

11. Protect your head.

Head injuries increase the risk of cognitive impairment in old age with concussions increasing risk by a factor of 10. Wear a helmet when it makes sense for the task and remain aware of your surroundings and the risk of head trauma.

12. Build social networks.

Life expectancy is increased in those with healthy social circles, so get out more often and make a commitment to becoming fully engaged in the community, especially if you're single.

Researchers at Wilkes University in Pennsylvania found that People who have regular sex take fewer sick days because they have higher levels of a certain antibody that defends the body against germs, viruses, and other intruders.

"Physical fitness is not only one of the most important keys to a healthy body, it is the basis of dynamic and creative intellectual activity."

– John F. Kennedy

Researchers at the Royal Edinburgh Hospital in Scotland conducted a long-term study of 3,500 people between the ages of 30 and 101 and found that regular sex may shave between four and seven years off your physical appearance, which leads me to believe that sex has no expiration date!

NEURO-CISE: SEXY SENIOR, DUO

Many make the mistake of thinking that the key to a spicier sex life at any age requires a different partner. This is especially true for couple's that have been together for a decade or more. It's assumed that everything has been tried and that you both know each other so well that there's no longer the element of surprise that makes a new partner so exciting.

This isn't true at all. Rediscovering a passionate connection between long-time partners can be as simple as making one single change or addition. As age settles in, we sometimes associate adventure, excitement and "sexual spiciness" with youth, but why should the young folks have all the fun? If you've earned your AARP card, you've earned your

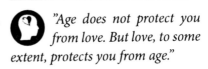

"Age does not protect you from love. But love, to some extent, protects you from age."

– *Jeanne Moreau*

right to the good life. It's only true that "you can't teach an old dog new tricks" if you keep on throwing the same bone in the same way.

Here's four ways to spice things up, regardless of age or limitations.

1. **Do something new together.** Sometimes the best way to add some excitement in the bedroom is to add some excitement in your life. And the newer the activity, the greater the increase of the feel good brain chemical dopamine, so don't settle for small new (a different restaurant) when you can go for big new (a weekend cooking or health retreat).

2. **Surprise your partner.** There's nothing sexier than a meaningful surprise. With couples that have been together a long time, a rut of routine can be easily remedied with a surprise. Don't wait for holidays, birthdays, and anniversaries to do the special things that say, "I still choose you."

3. **Switch it up.** After many years of sex with the same person, the actual act of making love can take on certain predictability. Something as simple as a different position (or a small change to a usual position) can add a healthy spark to the experience.

4. **Move it out.** Get out of the bedroom. There's a game many newlyweds play when they get into their first home where they make it a goal to have sex in EVERY room, including the yard, garage, shed, pool, and greenhouse. Maybe it's time for you and your partner to take a new tour of your old house.

Same Love, Differently Abled

The term "disabilities" covers a range of conditions including both congenital and acquired disabilities.

Approaching love, romance and intimacy can be especially challenging when dealing with disabilities. While the desire for love and intimacy is the same for everyone, finding romance is complicated by physical limitations and psychological challenges in a judgmental world.

First, the reality is that everyone is a little bit broken, and we all face disabilities in the bedroom at some time or another. That's the price of reaching adulthood. That is not to diminish the scope of challenges a person with disabilities may face, but it is hopefully a reminder that we all bring personal struggles into a relationship.

You might hold the belief that sex with disabilities is a hassle and burdensome. The truth is that sex with a disability can be better than sex without it. Hassle is about attitude. For one

"The only disability in life is a bad attitude."

–Scott Hamilton

person it may seem daunting to think creatively, maneuver, adjust, find alternative positions; for another it is a blessing. Navigating the myriad possibilities of how to be intimate allows people to escape routine sexual habits and keep things interesting. It supplies the opportunity to expand the meaning and experience of sex, and that is anything but a hassle!

In *The Ultimate Guide to Sex and Disability,* authors M. Kaufman, M.D., C. Silverberg, and F. Odette explain it like this: "Knowing when you get tired, realizing your limits, sensing when you're aroused by even the slightest physical cue—all are things that come with practice and are gifts that many others don't have. It's often assumed that disability creates a split between a person and their body because of the things they 'lost.' While this may happen to some, for many of us it's more true that learning to live without disabilities brings us closer to our bodies."

Below are some myths about sex and disabilities that need to be eliminated to make way for accurate knowledge, sexual skill building and differently-abled, erotic, intimate experiences.

- ♥ People with disabilities are asexual.

- ♥ If it isn't addressed, arousal won't happen.

- ♥ Their genitals don't work properly so they can't experience an orgasm.

- ♥ Only certain kinds of people hook up with disabled partners.

- ♥ The disability is more important than sexuality.

- ♥ People naturally know how to have sex, and if they don't, they shouldn't be having it.

- ♥ It is better not to risk reproduction.

- ♥ Sexuality is not part of healthcare.

- ♥ They are either innocent, too pure to have sex with or helpless victims, unable to have good sex.

- ♥ People with disabilities aren't at risk for sexual abuse.

The list above is 100% incorrect.

The hardest part of building a new relationship may be letting your guard down enough to allow for physical and sexual pleasure. Being hyper-aware of how you are "different" can hinder your ability to live fully in the moment. The single most important key in overcoming this challenge is the exact same key that remains vital to any and all successful relationships: communication.

Sex is not something you're born knowing how to do well. Human beings don't intrinsically know how to perform sexual acts, but rather require years of education and guidance on the subject. In my work with differently-abled clients, we focus on three basic fundamentals that are actually universal and not specific to differently-abled partners:

What Your Mind Says

First, be aware of what you're saying to yourself. One of the oldest clichés is "no one can love you until you learn to love yourself." Well, the reason that it's such an overly used phrase is that it's so very true. No matter what challenges life may have given you, before anyone will be able to truly love you, you have to be able to comfortably and confidently say three things:

1. I am worthy of love.

2. I am worthy of happiness.

3. I am worthy of respect.

4. I am worthy of great sex.

Yes, GREAT sex. Not "adequate." Not "fine." And certainly not "what the hell was that?" Say it with me now: I. Am. Worthy. Of. GREAT. Sex.

What Your Body Says

Not only is it important to pay attention to what your mind is telling you, you must listen and respect what your body is telling you. Your body is smarter than you are, so respect its signals, its red flags, and its orange cones that signal rough roads ahead. One of the exercises I recommend to my clients is to have a conversation with your body, including your most intimate parts. Give your body compliments and listen to your body's responses as it will always tell you the truth and serve you well if you treat it like you are madly in love with it, all of it, inside and out. If your sexual organs could talk, what would he or she say? And how would you respond?

While learning how to express yourself sexually, it's important to masturbate. Not only is it pleasurable in a way that doesn't involve being exposed to another person's eyes, but also it's very important learn or relearn one's body, to explore, and be creative. Masturbation is good for your health as a form of stress relief, it boosts your mood by releasing pleasure endorphins, acts as a natural sleep sedative, and can even relieve some forms of chronic pain such as headaches.

In order to tell someone how to touch you, you first have to know how you want to be touched.

What Your Mouth Says

Now that you've made peace with the inner world, it's time to express it to the outer world, most notably the ones you are inviting into your personal space. If you're going to get to someplace beautiful, you might have to start someplace ugly: the cold, hard truth.

Talk about your limitations. Explain your fears, your history and your desires. Being vulnerable is the ultimate sign of strength so you must be bravely fragile and say "I don't know what, if anything, will happen. I don't know where this journey will take me but if you're willing to try, I'm ready to go."

People often think of sexuality as those physical behaviors that occur between the sheets — specifically, sexual intercourse, but a range of other behaviors and paradigms also encompass the term sexuality. It is not about skill, but about honoring oneself and/or another individual(s) at that particular moment, similar to an interactive dance.

Yes, sexuality includes erotic fantasy, masturbation, procreation, and physical activity that can excite, (or is meant to excite) the genitals and/or the body's eroticism. But it also encompasses fetishism, turn-ons, and sexual orientation, which can be much more fluid than simply straight, bi or gay.

Sexuality is expressed in various ways that may include affection, tenderness, the desire to give as well as receive pleasure, compliments, companionship, tolerance, intimacy, verbal and non-verbal communication and love.

Sex and sexuality are a state of mind. All are natural; all are multifaceted, fluid and expansive. It is the integration of physical, emotional, intellectual and social aspects of an individual's personality.

Discover Your Own Happily Ever After

We get a lot of advice from the outside world on what our happiness should look like. Parents try to steer kids away from fruitless careers. Friends offer critiques of romantic partners. Strangers make judgments that can feel like standing in front of a firing squad. Ultimately though, we must embrace the life and love that brings us the most personal joy. We alone must stand in the middle of the life we live on a daily basis. Sometimes the days are easy and sometimes they're a battleground, so when you feel like you're fighting for survival, why not fight for a life you believe in? Creating a legacy that is truly an honest representation of who are you, without apology or remorse is an incredible thing to behold, and something we can all strive for.

It's impossible to live a life free of mistakes and challenges. And, really, why would you want that? Without mistakes there can be no forgiveness, without forgiveness there can be no love! It is a glorious feeling to overcome the obstacles that cause us to occasionally trip and fall. We learn, we grow, we evolve, we change, we love, we lose, and we love again.

As the errors of our ways come to light, it's important to remember this: if you've made a mistake, apologize for what you've done, never apologize for who you are.

Embrace the things that make you different. Enjoy the journey and all its unexpected detours. Find the path that makes your heart sing. Love the ones who inspire you to discover the best version of yourself. You're living the story of your life, so make sure that you're creating the best opportunity for a genuinely satisfying Happy Ending.

CHAPTER TEN
Happy Endings

My intention with this book is for you to have all the knowledge you need in order to live happily ever after. Isn't that what we all want? Through my personal journey and my work with others, I've learned that regardless of what life throws at us, we have the power to create a life that we love.

You already have the tools you need to accomplish this, whether you are looking for true love, to improve your current relationship, or just to learn how to love yourself. NeuroLoveology holds the key to mindful love and sex, which can transform your life.

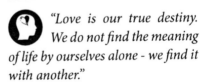 *"Love is our true destiny. We do not find the meaning of life by ourselves alone - we find it with another."*

– Thomas Merton

I urge you to use the lessons in this book to benefit your love life, whether it's how to overcome your past and move beyond what holds you back, or how to communicate successfully with your partner using his or her 'brain language.' You can rewrite the fairy tale that is your life and create your own happy ending - and you won't need a fairy godmother to make it happen because you have all the magic in your mind!

So embrace and commit to this acronym below from the word LOVE!

Learn

Optimize

Visualize

Empathize

Learn

Learn to love yourself just as you are. If necessary, you can "re-parent", giving yourself the love you didn't get as a child, and the love you always wanted. No matter what kind of childhood you've had, good or bad, it's time to take complete control of your life and accept who you are, idiosyncrasies and all, unconditionally.

NEURO-CISE: SELF-LOVE, SOLO

- ♥ What does your sub-conscious say when you look in the mirror? Every day, tell yourself that you have many lovable qualities, and list them.

- ♥ By loving yourself, you will attract a partner who balances you, not one who completes you. Give yourself an emotional, physical and appreciative compliment every day.

- ♥ Make a list of all your successes, big and small and then reward yourself generously.

- ♥ Make passionate love to yourself, just the way you want it.

- ♥ Forgive yourself for any negative self-talk and replace it with words of love.

Whether you're looking for love, building love or trying to rekindle love, the same rule applies: you will only get what you are willing to give. If what you want is to be fully accepted with all your idiosyncrasies, you must practice compassion and open-mindedness. Regardless of the media messages to the contrary, there is no such thing as perfection. That is an impossible goal that carries with it only disappointment, fear and anxiety. Our differences are our strengths, not our weaknesses, but only if respect comes first. This includes self-respect.

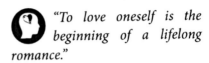

"To love oneself is the beginning of a lifelong romance."

– Oscar Wilde

While it's necessary to clarify what you need from other people, it's equally important to be able to find the areas where you can compromise. Successful relationships are based on the partner's abilities to adapt to the changes and challenges that come over the course of a lifetime. While many of the core elements will remain the same, people change as life lessons and opportunities come along. Like love, life is not static. It ebbs and flows. It has moments of ease and moments of struggle. How this evolution is faced determines its success or failure. Regardless of what comes along, the solution can be both simple and difficult. But above all else, choose kindness.

"Books can inspire you to love yourself more, but by listening to, writing out, or verbally expressing your feelings you are actually doing it."

– Dr. John Gray

Kindness can sometimes be confused for weakness, which couldn't be further from the truth. Kindness is at the base of forgiveness, apology, respect, and love. All of those things take incredible strength and fortitude. Making the choice to be kind isn't the same as choosing to be passive. It's about being honest but respectful.

Love Is A Choice

Before you can examine and explore the outer world, you must take inventory of the inner world so you are clear about what tools make up the toolbox of your life. You must choose to see yourself clearly, without shame. Look in the mirror. Look

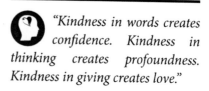

"Kindness in words creates confidence. Kindness in thinking creates profoundness. Kindness in giving creates love."

– Lao Tzu

at your face. Whatever has happened, that is the face of a survivor. That is a face of love. That is the face that can change the world. See it. Accept it. Embrace it. Free it.

Neuropsychiatrists have shown that when you accept and love yourself, it helps the prefrontal cortex to build a clear path to overcoming challenges in order to reach your goals.

Love is a series of conscious choices and remaining mindful of these choices is the key to its success.

Who?

Who are you right now? Regardless of goals and dreams, you can't get there without a clear picture of your starting point. Otherwise you may be blind to the stumbling blocks that will repeatedly, subconsciously keep you from the life and love that you desire.

What?

What are you willing to do to make your dream life a reality? Be honest, because only in this honesty will you realize your strengths and weaknesses. Additionally, if you come to accept that you're not able or willing to do something that is required for making the goal a reality, it will free you to adjust or release the goal in order to make way for one that is attainable.

When?

When will you take action to make the next chapter of your life a reality? The answer should always be "now", even if the action seems miniscule. The tiniest shift or movement can create a 'butterfly effect' that completely alters your path. If you're not familiar, the butterfly effect is a concept in chaos theory wherein the smallest change can have enormous consequences. A butterfly that flaps its wings in Brazil can lead to a windstorm in Chicago. Likewise, cleaning your bedroom as if to impress your partner (even if you don't yet have one) may lead to just such a guest.

Where?

Where are your roadblocks and how can you move them, destroy them or work around them? Some are facts (age, children, parents, illness, physical limitations) but many are life lessons that have created insecurities, doubts, and fears that underscore a false message of self-worth. While you cannot change the fact that you are a 40-year-old with a thrice-divorced track record, you can change your perception of this situation and foster a completely new approach to relationships.

Why?

Why is your current situation the way it is? Can you answer that question and take 100% of the responsibility? Obviously you're not fully responsible for everything that has ever happened in your life since situations and events do come along that are beyond your individual control. However, you are 100% responsible for your *response* to these circumstances.

How?

How can your past become your wings and not your anchor? Life is full of extraordinary lessons that test us on a daily basis. If you look back on your life, how can you find the lessons of yesterday that create a foundation for a better tomorrow? Poor decisions made in the past often leave us with regret that can keep us from believing we are worthy of the happiness we desire. Mistakes get made. That is the price of admission for the ride of life. But just because they were made in the past doesn't mean they will be made again.

NEURO-CISE: EMBODIMENT, SOLO

Dr. Stella Resnick, psychologist, psychotherapist, and author of *The Heart of Desire* and *The Pleasure Zone*, specializes in embodiment exercises that can help you to identify blocked emotions that are affecting you physically.

Here are some exercises recommended by Dr. Resnick to help release negative emotions, some of which may have been planted years ago, that have culminated into physical distress.

With your eyes closed, scan your body and notice any tension you may feel in your emotional center, that area of your body between your head and your pelvis.

Head

Start with the top of your head, forehead, eyes, cheeks, mouth and jaw, breathe deeply and see if any of these areas are tight. Tension here is usually a sign of mental stress, negative thinking, and a tendency to overanalyze situations and to try to figure things out. A tight mouth and jaw can be a sign of anger.

Throat

Take a deep sigh and tune into your throat and see if you have a grip or lump in your throat. A grip is often a sign of anxiety; a lump usually has to do with feeling sad.

Chest

Take another deep sigh and check your chest. See if there is a weight on your chest, a band around your chest, or a grip in the center of the chest. A weight suggests you're feeling hurt or disappointed. A grip or band usually indicates anxiety.

Diaphragm

From there, take a sigh and feel for any knot in your diaphragm. A knot here is likely a sign of guilt, feelings of responsibility and obligation.

Belly
Check your belly and see if you have a knot or butterflies. A knot can be tied to fear or anger. A feeling of butterflies usually means dread about the future.

Pelvis
Finally, take a deep sigh and make a mental note of any tension in your genitals, thighs, or buttocks, which often indicates feelings of shame.

This exercise is also known as "self-regulation of stress" and it can be very helpful even after only a minute or two of practice.

Give Kindness Away
If you hand someone a dollar as an act of kindness, they become one dollar richer, but you don't automatically become one dollar poorer. Their gratitude will warm you, and when the day comes that you need a dollar, it will be there. The concept of "give first" can be a difficult one to comprehend in the me-me-me society we live in.

How can I suggest that you feed someone when it is you that is starving? I'm not talking about actual food, but the nourishment of kindness and love. How can I say that if you want love that you should give love first? Because the giving is part of the getting. You cannot have one without the other. It is the flow of energy between people that sustains us. Sometimes this energy is found in sharing a loaf of bread or a bottle of water. Other times, this energy is a hug, a smile, a compliment, holding the door for a stranger, helping an elderly person reach something on a high shelf in a store. We GET by GIVING.

So, if you're single and looking for love, start giving love to everyone you meet. No, no, no, not quickies with every stranger on the block, but genuine kindness. It can have surprising effects because it is so rare in the detached, impersonal world we live in. Your act of kindness may be seen by the next love of your life and inspire them to say hello.

If you're in a relationship that's floundering, figure out how to love your partner better. Listen for the clues as to what they feel is lacking. If you're not sure what they need, give them what you need. If you wish your partner were more romantic, buy them

> *"Giving connects two people, the giver and the receiver, and this connection gives birth to a new sense of belonging."*
>
> – *Dr. Deepak Chopra*

flowers or surprise them with a special date. You cannot demand that someone else lower their guard without first lowering your own.

We've all seen acts of kindness on the news and in Internet posts that lift our spirits. Usually they're billed as "Stories to restore your faith in humanity" or something similar. How tragic that the underlying message is, "Yes, life usually sucks and people are awful but look here, sometimes they surprise you by being compassionate!" Many times acts of heroism are portrayed as gigantic, epic, and life risking, like running into a burning building to save children. No denying that is truly extraordinary. But many of us are trapped in the burning buildings of our minds and it's no less lifesaving when someone sees that and runs in to save the day. Why not practice kindness and become one of those news stories?

There are countless stories of romantic situations where one partner is ready to give up on trying to fix what feels broken when suddenly their mate surprises them in a way that makes them feel respected, understood and seen. Positive

> *"Kindness is more important than wisdom, and the recognition of that is the beginning of wisdom."*
>
> – *Dr. Theodore Rubin*

shifts can happen with the simplest of actions.

These actions typically utilize the same fundamental elements: respect, communication, passion, trust and friendship. In a nutshell, kindness.

Linda Graham is a marriage and family therapist and author of *Bouncing Back: Rewiring Your Brain for Maximum Resilience and Well-Being*. She writes in her book, "As you remember experiencing a moment of kindness, your brain lights up all the networks of that memory; the visual image, the emotions, and the body sensations, as well as the thoughts and beliefs. You convey the entire experience to your partner through your facial expressions, body language and tone of voice, as well as your words. As your partner attunes to you, mirror neurons in his brain pick up the nonverbal signals of your inner experience and begin to register in his brain as his own inner experience of your inner experience."

Dr. Stella Resnick believes these mirror neurons have healing powers as well. "In essence, two loving people can silently transmit information back and forth through eye contact as well as touch that can adjust each other's heart rate, hormone levels, disease fighting blood cells, and more. This is called entrainment or neural synchrony."

Optimize

Not only is it important to optimize all of your assets in order to ensure the best outcome in any situation, it's also important to optimize your outlook by remaining positive and hopeful.

According to studies at Yale University, a positive attitude is actually more important for living a longer life than even low blood pressure, regular exercise, good weight and even a smoke free environment. A positive attitude is more important than success or failure, so look for the positive in everything and everyone.

RVM, author of *Power Your Life With PEP, Discover the Secret of Thinking and Living Positively All the Time* describes attitude as "the raw material that produces thought. The magical ingredient that creates attitude

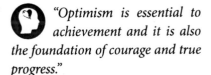

"Optimism is essential to achievement and it is also the foundation of courage and true progress."

– *Nicholas M. Butler*

is emotion." He calls *PEP Positive Energy Power:* "It is the power that can lead us to a positive destiny."

NEURO-CISE: OPTIMISM, SOLO

♥ You can train yourself to find the positive in everything and everyone by turning on your personal "Happy Face." Visualize a time in your life when you were happy and hold that thought. Our thoughts control our lives and we have the power to change our thoughts at any time or place, so for your health's sake, take control.

♥ A positive attitude is contagious, releases pleasure endorphins and de-stresses the body, so be sure to call friends and family just to wish them well.

♥ In a relationship, imagine that your partner is wearing a crown and think about what would you say or do to make them feel like a king or queen.

Look for something positive in your past, even if it is simply a positive lesson from a difficult experience. Some of life's greatest struggles lead to the most promising outcomes. All of us somewhere along the way have been hurt by someone - a partner, friend, teacher, parent or even ourselves through negative self-talk - and by examining these negative experiences we can find positive aspects to focus on. The key is learning to see a breakdown as a breakthrough.

Every thought affects the brain, and placing focus on negative thoughts slows down its ability to function. Conversely, positive thinking balances serotonin and releases oxytocin, which supports a healthy sense of self and peak brain function. Happy thoughts also generate brain growth, especially in the prefrontal cortex, which is the only part of the brain that controls emotions and behaviors.

Turn Up the Volume On Your Life

The life you want is going to take some serious action on your part. The world is full of people making wish lists but taking no actual steps to make those things happen. You must put your hands on the wheel and turn it even just a little bit in order to alter the path that you're on. No situation can improve without your involvement; it can only stay the same or get worse. Why not help ensure that the change is a positive one?

NEURO-CISE: BE BOLD, SOLO

Do something bold. Not HUGE bold, like quit your job, jump the cute guy behind the coffee counter or show up at your partner's office with nothing under your coat but your flesh. Just something small bold,

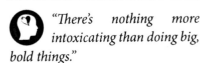 *"There's nothing more intoxicating than doing big, bold things."*

– Jason Kilar

perhaps something that no one even realizes is bold except for you. Talk to the human resources department about the requirements for a different position. Say hello to the guy at the coffee shop by using his name, if you know it. Join a dating service or singles group. If you surprise yourself, even subtly, you will ignite an adrenaline rush that reminds you that you're a living, breathing creature capable of greatness and deserving of love.

Be A Truth Seeker

Learn to see the facts of a situation for what they are, and don't confuse them with your feelings. In previous chapters I've discussed how our brains react to certain triggers, creating emotional responses that don't always help us to interpret events clearly. Armed with that information, your control over a given situation is greatly improved.

Snap judgment, misinterpretation, and fear are the cause of more emotional damage than actual spiteful intentions. As the saying goes, "the truth shall set you free", which is never more accurately applied than when we're looking to resolve conflict. With honesty and understanding we have the potential to heal. Respond with logic and open-mindedness when confronted with an emotional challenge, and reap the rewards of focusing on the truth, rather than your own 'story'. A few deep breaths can go a long way toward protecting what might be otherwise destroyed with hasty remarks. It's called the 'high road'. It might be less travelled, but there are way fewer potholes!

Enjoy The Journey

Remember Daniel Kahneman's breakthrough discovery that the brain ultimately remembers only two aspects of an event: the emotional peak and the end. This is important as you move forward in your life, especially in your romantic relationships. In order to build a deep connection, you must pay attention to the emotional flow of events.

We live in a culture that is focused on the "big finish", which does have certain logic to it. I mean, imagine if a fireworks show started with its biggest, brightest, most dramatic and colorful display and then followed with a series of increasing less impressive fireworks. Better yet, imagine starting sex with the best orgasm of your life and then trying to maintain interest in the twenty minutes of playfulness that follows. Obviously we want to save the best for last because the anticipation of a great finale heightens the joy of the journey. However, we need to remember to drop some "hints of greatness" along the way.

Oftentimes we associate the emotional peak with the end, but that's not always the case and can, in fact, undermine a positive experience if the emotional peak is negative. If

"Love is not a feeling. Love is an action, an activity."

– Dr. M. Scott Peck

a date ends with a marriage proposal, that is definitely memorable, but if dinner was interrupted with an argument that included cruel remarks, that is just as memorable and could quite possibly change the answer to the big question.

NEURO-CISE: HIGH PEAKS, SOLO

Tap into your most positive peak memories to experience pleasure by closing your eyes and recalling a moment when you felt like you were on top of the world. It could be a birthday celebration, wedding, graduation, getting a raise, having a great date, your first kiss or orgasm. This powerful neuro-cise results in reprogramming the subconscious mind and flooding your body with feel good endorphins, as your brain doesn't know the difference between whether you are thinking or experiencing your peak moments.

NEURO-CISE: HIGH PEAKS, DUO

Look for ways to increase high points throughout the course of a romantic journey. This is as important for a first coffee date that lasts thirty minutes as it is for a marriage that lasts thirty years. Pay attention to the end goal and make reaching it a priority, but pay equal attention to the journey and constantly be on the lookout for ways to incorporate emotional high peaks along the way. In other words, make every romantic connection a memorable one, whether it's setting the scene for romance by incorporating all of your senses or taking turns to create fantasy date nights that you'll be talking about into your twilight years. In the end, nothing is as important as the beautiful memories that we have created with the ones we love.

Visualize

Visualizing is not the same thing as daydreaming, though they may start from the same place. They both require imagination, but only visualization requires action as well. By imagining a goal in every detail with great focus, you begin the process of shifting your path towards realizing that goal. The brain doesn't distinguish between what you imagine and what you experience.

If you think about riding a rollercoaster, closing your eyes and imagining every turn, rise and drop as if you're sitting in one of the cars, your heart rate will increase, your hands will tighten and you will experience the body jolts of adrenaline that match almost exactly the same physical response to actually experiencing that ride. The same goes for creating shifts in personal awareness. If you are insecure but you visualize how you imagine it would feel to walk through life with confidence, your brain will start behaving as if this is true. You will stand taller, your shoulders will slip back, you will raise your eyes and head.

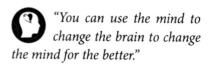

"You can use the mind to change the brain to change the mind for the better."

– *Dr. Rick Hanson*

This is the strength behind affirmations. If you say something repeatedly, *even if you don't yet believe it,* your subconscious mind will start to live as if it is true and slowly what you wish will become reality.

For many, visualizing a life that they don't yet have seems depressing. *Why would I want to focus on what I don't have?* That's not the point of visualization at all. The important word missing from this question is "yet." Why would I want to focus on what I don't YET have? Because it prepares you for the having. It imbeds in the mind an ability to deal with whatever may come with reaching a goal and it reduces some of the anxiety of the unknown which, in many cases, creates a wall of fear between where we are and where we want to be. By visualizing, we can test out scenarios and imagine how questions and challenges might be faced and overcome. We begin to see how we would function in the life we want, and that allows us to move into that life with calmness and self-awareness.

Dr. Charlotte Tomaino is a former nun who studies the field of neuroplasticity with over 30 years of clinical experience as a neuropsychologist. She writes in her book, *Awakening the Brain,* "Your intention focuses your brain on why you want to build that neural network and sustains your effort through all the mistakes you make until you reach automaticity. Yes, if you persist, it will become an automatic skill. You will reinvent who you are. Because I persisted, I am now a neuropsychologist and a writer, and a whole new world for sharing this

"The brain is a use it or lose it organ."

- *Dr. Charlotte Tomaino*

information is available to me to offer it to you. To access the power of neuroplasticity to enhance the mental functions of your brain, persistence is essential."

One of the tools of visualization is intention, which can help to access right brain functioning and dominance.

NEURO-CISE: AUTOBIOGRAPHY, SOLO

One visualization technique that can help formulate ideas and a game plan is to imagine yourself five years from now, writing about the things that have taken place between now and then. Instead of thinking "this is what I want to do", envision that you have already done it and you are looking back from a place of success, describing in detail how your life has changed. What does your life look like five years from now? Don't think about a huge achievement or event, just imagine an average day. How does the day start? Where are you? Who is lying beside you? What activities fill your day in a way that leaves you feeling comfortable, safe and content? If you can see and describe that day in great detail, it can instigate in the brain a desire to make that a reality and you may find that a game plan starts to formulate and opportunities may suddenly arise that seem to support that goal.

We previously discussed the use of creating a mission statement for a relationship, outlining needs and goals for the life you are building together. This is an equally important exercise for a single person. We are taught not to be selfish, and that life and love is about compromise and giving. These things are obviously important, but no less important than recognizing your own deal breakers and the things you need to be given in order to feel comfortable in a relationship.

NEURO-CISE: LIFE CHART, SOLO

RVM created a Future Introspection Life Chart with 12 thought provoking questions that can help you to conceive, believe and achieve the kind of future that you want to live.

1. What are my 5 priorities of life in the near future?

_____

_____

_____

_____

_____

2. I hope to live until I am _____

3. What is missing in my life _____

4. My biggest problem is _____

5. My unfulfilled dreams and desires are

_____

_____

_____

_____

6. What 5 things make me happiest?

_____

_____

_____

_____

_____

7. Money

(a) Do I need more? _____

(b) How much more? _____

(c) For what? _____

(d) What I plan to do with my money after my life?

_____

_____

8. What I want my life to be

(a) Next year _____

(b) After 5 years _____

(c) After 10 years _____

(d) After 20 years _____

9. What changes do I need to make for my health?

_____

_____

_____

_____

10. What changes do I seek to make on how I spend my time?

_____

_____

_____

_____

11. What are the changes I must make for me to get to where I want to go?

_____

_____

_____

_____

12. Resolutions I am making today

_____

_____

_____

_____

NEURO-CISE: DREAM LIST, SOLO

When it comes to relationships, you can also create your wish list, drawing to you the partner you desire. But beware that often our list of requirements is extensive and we can paint ourselves into a corner of disappointment by seeking a partner that matches 100% of this list. Ultimately, however, this list is much more flexible than we realize. The following exercise will help you become more open to different types of people by challenging your sense of what is a deal-breaker. You can broaden your dating reach by letting go of that rigid definition of your future partner.

1. Make a list of twenty traits that you believe would make up your ideal mate. Include everything: appearance ("brown hair"), personality ("dry sense of humor"), skills ("good cook"), and profession ("doctor"). You can include more than 20 but it's a good number to set as a goal.

2. Now review your list carefully AND CUT IT IN HALF. Look at each list item and decide if it is a request or a requirement and cross off those items that are not absolute necessities.

3. Do this again. Yes, cut the list in half again using the same

critique. Take two items on the list and place them side-by-side. Consider which one would be more difficult to live without and save that one while deleting the other one.

4. If you started with a list longer than 20, continue examining the list and comparing traits until you are down to five.

This exercise has been quite eye opening for several of my clients because a list that started with a lot of physical attributes was quickly reduced to a series of personality attributes. We all have a physical type that we are

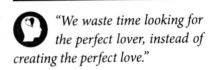

"We waste time looking for the perfect lover, instead of creating the perfect love."

– Tom Robbins

drawn to but in long-term relationships, we gradually begin to see our partners less for how they look and more for how they make us feel, so clarifying your list can help you see potential relationships more clearly.

NEURO-CISE: COIN TOSS, SOLO

No, I'm not telling you to leave the fate of your life up to a coin toss, but there is something interesting to be discovered in pretending to do so.

Let's use the exercise above as an example. There are two traits between which you are trying to decide. Assign each of them a side of coin and then make the toss. With the coin in the air, you will likely realize immediately that your thought becomes "please let it land on ..." When it comes down to only two options and you are forced to make a choice, there is always a preference, even if the divide is invisible to the human eye. The answer is not in how the coin actually lands but in how you want it to land.

Empathize

Empathy is a positive habit you can cultivate to improve your life and the lives of everyone near and dear to you.

Neuroscientists have identified a 10-section "empathy circuit" in our brains which, if damaged, can inhibit our ability to understand what other people are feeling.

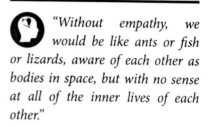

"Without empathy, we would be like ants or fish or lizards, aware of each other as bodies in space, but with no sense at all of the inner lives of each other."

– Dr. Rick Hanson

Empathy lights up two main areas in the brain, the insula and cingulate cortex, both of which are part of the emotional and physical regions. These areas, plus mirror neurons, produce recreations of the other person's experience inside your own brain so that you can feel yourself "in their shoes."

It's also important to learn how to have self-empathy. As humans, we live with divided minds. We are able to look at our own thoughts and decisions and judge them just as easily as we can judge the choices made by other people. In fact, we are likely more critical of our own behaviors than we are of someone else's. A mistake made to us may be easier to forgive than if we were to make the same mistake to someone else.

We must learn to treat ourselves with the same kindness that we offer to the ones we love. We have to be understanding and allow for errors because it is in these mistakes that personal growth happens.

In the game of love and sex, you risk getting hurt when you reveal your emotional and sexual vulnerabilities. But if you don't risk getting hurt, you won't learn how to give and receive true love or sexual intimacy. So here are some steps to help you fall in love and have great sex.

NEURO-CISE: EMPATHY, DUO

Happiness guru Martin Seligman identifies empathy as a key character strength that can enhance life satisfaction.

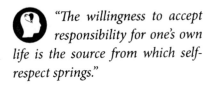

"The willingness to accept responsibility for one's own life is the source from which self-respect springs."

– Joan Didion

♥ Have empathetic conversations by listening to others and responding with your supportive emotions for mutual understanding.

♥ Practice empathy with people whose beliefs are different than yours and try to step into their shoes to understand their thinking.

♥ Create empathy with your partner by fully accepting his or her emotions and perceptions and validate them with a nurturing hug.

NEURO-CISE: EMPATHY, SOLO

♥ Start by treating yourself as if you are madly in love with you. That means valuing and pleasuring yourself, rewarding and accepting yourself, validating and loving yourself unconditionally. Look, if you don't have a great relationship with yourself, it's not going to work with another person.

♥ Next, be willing to let someone go when the bad outweighs the good. Say "No" to people making demands on your valuable time if they don't give you the attention, appreciation, respect or sexual satisfaction that you need to make you happy.

♥ On the other hand, if you have great sexual chemistry with someone who knows how to turn you on, but doesn't fulfill your emotional needs, don't deprive yourself of mind-blowing orgasms. There's no rule that says you have to be in love to have great sex or that having great sex will destroy the possibility of having true love.

The greatest irony of having sex without love or love without sex is that most people focus on what is missing as opposed to holding on to what they have. Love won't hurt when your heart is filled with gratitude and you feel complete as a person with or without a partner.

Go On Now, Be Brave

Make gratitude a more integral part of your life. Sometimes the simplest, most eloquent way to reach a person's heart is to say "thank you." There is no better way to communicate appreciation than through compliments, so make them a daily ritual. Saying something meaningful, appreciative and caring to someone special helps cement your relationship with them. It's a way to build and maintain a positive relationship that grows and lasts. Take the time to tell people what qualities make them so special and important to your life.

Dr. Daniel Amen, psychiatrist and author of over 30 books including *Sex on the Brain: 12 Lessons to Enhance your Love Life* discovered that gratitude literally changes the brain chemistry in a positive way, especially in the areas of the frontal lobes and cerebellum. Increased blood flow in these areas results in better decisions, focus and judgment. The pituitary gland releases feel good endorphins that flood the brain and body with an overall sense of mental and physical pleasure.

Don't forget to pamper yourself. Decide what it is that gives you the most pleasure. Is it eating dessert? Watching a romantic or scary movie? Getting a massage or pedicure? Taking a nap in the middle of the day? Reading a book? Having a picnic or going dancing? You decide and then put it into action. In order to love yourself you must consider yourself worthy of rewards.

It pays to take your needs seriously. So, take this opportunity to do special things for yourself that you may have postponed. Get to know you better and romance yourself because you deserve it. Any love you experience beyond that will only be greater.

NEURO-CISE: GRATITUDE, SOLO

Think of three things that you are grateful for and write them down every day in a gratitude journal, on your computer or even on index cards. Researchers did a controlled study where participants carried out this gratitude exercise every day for a week and they found that they were happier and less depressed. The results were published in the American Psychological Association APA PsycNET.

NEURO-CISE: GRATITUDE, DUO

Text your partner a sexy gratitude message: "Thank u for being so sexy." "I'm so grateful for your love." If you want to, write a love letter of gratitude by letting your partner know how much you appreciate having him or her in your life, it can make your love life even deeper.

The Network of Love

The network of love includes the emotional side of the brain where you'll find the limbic system that is responsible for how we express what we feel. The logical side of the brain on the other hand, determines reasoning to help us judge if a person is going to complement

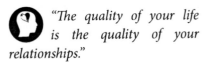

"The quality of your life is the quality of your relationships."

– Anthony Robbins

us by being a good partner. The impulse relay station in the network of love is the thalamus located in the core of the brain, which plays a major role in regulating sensory awareness and arousal.

Neurological research has revealed that love is a complex emotion that activates twelve different areas of the brain that are responsible for motivation, emotion, attention and memory. With brain imaging of people who are deeply in love, areas of the brain that are associated with reward, desire, pleasure and euphoria are highly active.

Love is not to be taken for granted, so treat it with respect, both the love you have to give and the love you are lucky enough to receive. We live in a time when giving up quickly is far too easy. The divorce rate is an embarrassment to the concept of love. What might be different if it weren't so easy to quit? I have witnessed marriages where the couple is adamant about their commitment to marriage, but they have defined it as settling for unhappiness. While divorce might be seen as "giving up," so is the choice to remain unhappy! Unless you are part of an arranged marriage, the two of you came together by choice. You were drawn to each other so fully that you made the mutual decision to commit to building a life together. If the kindness, friendship and respect were there once upon a time, they are still there, hiding under the layers of pain, doubt, miscommunication, and silent fear. The work to uncover them again may seem daunting, but isn't it worth it to fight for a chance to make our lives better?

Love is one of life's greatest pleasures. Let yourself experience it in all its glory. Do the work. Enrich the relationships you have. Learn about your partner on a daily basis. Test yourself constantly. Show more kindness today than you did yesterday. Boldly be exactly who are you. The world needs more beauty and nothing is more beautiful than love.

Be brave enough to let someone in, because only when we're truly seen are we truly free.

NEURO-CISES INDEX

FURTHER READING

The Art of Everyday Ecstasy
Author: Margot Anand

Awakening the Brain
Author: Dr. Charlotte Tomaino

Bouncing Back:
Rewiring Your Brain for Maximum Resilience and Wellbeing
Author: Linda Graham

Brain Rules
Author: Dr. John Medina

Brains and Realities
Author: Jay Alfred

Buddha's Brain:
The Practical Neuroscience of Happiness, Love and Wisdom
Author: Rick Hanson

Conquer Prostate Cancer:
How Medicine, Faith, Love and Sex Can Renew Your Life
Author: Rabbi Ed Weinberg, Ed.D, DD

Craving for Ecstasy: The Consciousness and Chemistry of Escape
Author: Dr. Harvey Milkman and Dr. Stanley Sunderwirth

Daring to Live Fully
Author: Marelisa Fabrega

The Enlightened Brain
Author: Rick Hanson

The Female Brain
Author: Loann Brizendine

Forgive for Good
Author: Dr. Fred Luskin

The G-Spot and Other Discoveries About Human Sexuality
Author: Beverly Whipple

Hardwiring Happiness
Author: Dr. Rick Hanson

*The Healing Power of Sound: Recovering
from Life-Threatening Illness Using, Sound, Voice and Music*
Author: Dr. Mitchell Gaynor

The Heart of Desire
Author: Stella Resnick

Love Addict: Sex, Romance and Other Dangerous Drugs
Author: Ethlie Ann Vare

Love Lessons: A Guide to Transforming Relationships
Author: Dr. Brenda Wade

*Lust, Anger, Love: Understanding Sexual Addiction
and the Road to Road to Healthy Intimacy*
Author: Maureen Canning

The Male Brain
Author: Loann Brizendine

Mars & Venus Collide
Author: Dr. John Gray

Men Are from Mars, Women Are from Venus
Author: Dr. John Gray

The Mommy Brain: How Motherhood Makes Us Smarter
Author: Katherine Ellison

The Now Effect
Author: Dr. Elisha Goldstein

Organize Your Mind, Organize Your Life
Author: Margaret Moore

The One Thing Holding You Back:
Unleashing the Power of Emotional Connection
Author: Raphael Cushnir

Opposites Attract
Author: Rebecca Cutter

The Owner's Manual of the Brain
Author: Dr. Pierce J. Howard

The Pleasure Zone
Author: Stella Resnick

Power your Life with PEP,
Discover the Secret of Thinking and Living Positively All the Time
Author: RVM

The Science of Kissing: What Our Lips Are Telling Us
Author: Sheril Kirshenbaum

Sex on the Brain: 12 Lessons to Enhance You Love Life
Author: Daniel Amen

The Sexy Little Book of Sex Games
Author: Dr. Ava Cadell

She Comes First: The Thinking Man's Guide to Pleasing a Woman
Author: Kerner

Slice of the Beloved
Author: Gurutej Khalsa

Thanks! How the New Science of Gratitude Can Make You Happier
Author: Robert Emmons, PhD

Thinking, Fast and Slow
Author: Daniel Kahneman

Thriving with Heart Disease
Author: Dr. Wayne Sotile

The Ultimate Guide to Sex and Disability
Author: M. Kaufman, M.D, C. Silverberg, and F. Odette

The Willpower Instinct
Author: Dr. Kelly McGonigal

Why God Won't Go Away: Brain Science and Biology of Belief
Author: Dr. Andrew Newberg and Dr. Eugene d'Aquili

Your Brain at Work
Author: Dr. David Rock

COACHING AND COUNSELING

Dr. Ava lectures around the globe about finding love, enriching relationships, creating romance, enhancing intimacy, and expanding sexuality for a more fulfilling life. She speaks from personal experience, her private counseling practice and Loveology University, inspiring others to find and maintain their passion. To learn more about Dr. Ava's lecture series, private practice or her Loveology University, please visit

www.avacadell.com

CPSIA information can be obtained at www.ICGtesting.com
Printed in the USA
BVOW04s2030190314

348180BV00002B/20/P